AF412783

Advances in Radiation Therapy

Progress in Tumor Research

Vol. 44

Series Editors

Rolf A. Stahel Zurich
Solange Peters Lausanne

Advances in Radiation Therapy

Volume Editors

M. Guckenberger Zurich
S.E. Combs Munich
D. Zips Tübingen

24 figures, 20 in color, and 4 tables, 2018

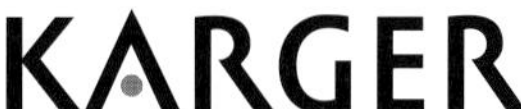

Basel · Freiburg · Paris · London · New York · Chennai · New Delhi ·
Bangkok · Beijing · Shanghai · Tokyo · Kuala Lumpur · Singapore · Sydney

Preface

Clinically relevant progress has been made in the diagnosis and treatment of cancer in recent decades; however, this progress varies substantially between cancer types and between countries with variable access to health care resources. Five-year survival rates have improved beyond 50% for breast cancer and colon cancer, whereas lung cancer is associated with poor survival of <20% and only very little progress has been made with overall survival improvements of 2–4% in Europe and North America [1].

Advances in biological disease characterization has accelerated progress in many cancer types. In non-small cell lung cancer (NSCLC) and melanoma – previously associated with a devastating prognosis in metastatic state – patients with an activating driver mutation (EGRF, ALK, BRAF) achieve long-term survival when treated with targeted drugs or, since recently, with immune checkpoint inhibition. The field of radiation oncology has advanced in parallel with the progress in medical oncology and has improved the precision of cancer treatment and outcome for our cancer patients. Radiation oncology is characterized by the interaction of technology and cancer and patient biology, and by the interdisciplinary and multi-professional practice of cancer treatment and research. Consequently, progress has been achieved in the 3 distinct fields of: (a) radiobiology and combined modality treatment, (b) radiotherapy technology, and (c) particle therapy [2, 3].

Better understanding of radiation and cancer biology is a major driving force of innovation towards better radiotherapy [4]. For radiation oncology, the main areas of ongoing development include combinations with immunotherapy, targeting of the tumour microenvironment, and integration of imaging biomarkers for individualized treatments [3]. These areas are covered in dedicated sections and reflect the current status and future perspectives. While checkpoint inhibition leads to unprecedented and sometimes longlasting remission rates in some types of cancer, such as malignant melanoma, it is becoming more and more evident that the majority of cancers are resistant to immunotherapy. Resistance to immunotherapy either from the beginning (primary resistance) or later during the course of treatment after an initial response (secondary or acquired resistance) is a remaining challenge and an area of intense research [5]. Conceptually, one strategy to overcome resistance is the use of combinatorial approaches of different immunotherapies with other treatment modalities, such as radiation, chemotherapy, and targeted agents. Better understanding of immunotherapy and radiation biology might result in the definition of a new role for radiotherapy. Interestingly, mechanisms of resistance to immunotherapies include a suppressive tumour microenvironment and tumour hypoxia, i.e., well-established factors of resistance to radiotherapy and targeted agents. This functional link may suggest novel approaches, such imaging strategies and therapeutic manipulations, leading to better prediction and treatment adaptation of rational combinations in the future [6].

Radiation oncology has participated in the rapid progress made in computational sciences and biomedical engineering. As a consequence, radiation therapy is planned and delivered in a very different way compared to the standards of the last century. As a non-invasive treatment, radiation oncology is an imaging-based and imaging-driven treatment modality. Multimodality imaging for target and organ-at-risk definition using CT, MRI, and PET imaging has become the standard of care in many cancer sites and has improved accuracy and reproducibility. For example, FDG-PET is a mandatory component of NSCLC staging [7] and MRI-based prostate segmentation is a mandatory component of radical radiotherapy planning for prostate cancer [8]. Functional imaging for biological disease characterization has been explored for many years but is still at a research stage and has not yet become a standard of care [9]. Recent research has evaluated the potential of quantitative computational image analysis for the comprehensive characterization of medical images [10, 11], a methodology called radiomics. Radiotherapy treatment planning is today using intensity-modulated techniques in routine clinical practice, which has improved dosimetric treatment characteristics and, subsequently, clinical outcome [12, 13]. Current progress is aiming to identify the optimal patient-tailored individual treatment plan with improved accuracy and reliability; different solutions have been proposed using, for example, libraries of previous treatments, multi-criteria optimization, and Pareto navigation [14, 15]. Continuous re-assessment of cancer biology and target geometry, and its integration into treatment by adaptive re-planning, is currently being explored in particular in the context of hybrid devices of combined linear accelerators and MRI [16]. Stereotactic radiotherapy has been practiced for decades for the treatment of benign and malignant brain tumours, and technological advances of highly conformal treatment planning and image-guided treatment delivery has allowed its transfer to the body part in the form of stereotactic body radiotherapy (SBRT) [17]. Today, SBRT is the standard of care for medically inoperable early-stage NSCLC [18] and outcomes appear similar to results achieved by the gold standard of surgery [19]. The characteristics of SBRT to achieve very high rates of local tumour control in a few non-invasive and ambulatory treatment sessions is the rational to explore its potential in many other cancer types. SBRT appears highly promising not only in early cancer stages, but in particular in the stage of oligometastatic disease, when integrated into and combined with effective systemic treatment [20–22].

Particle therapy represents one of the most promising improvements in radiation oncology in recent years. Particle therapy has distinct physical properties leading to a reduction of integral dose compared to photons. On top of that, ion beam therapy has to be divided into protons with almost comparable biological effect to photons, and carbon ions or other heavier charged particles with an increased relative biological effectiveness. So, on the one hand there is proton radiotherapy, where indications are comparable to photons, and on the other hand there is high-LET particle beams, where clinical trials are necessary to determine the tumours that are most sensitive to them. The rationale for proton beams is mainly reducing the dose exposure to normal tissue and for carbon ions treating radioresistant tumours, such as slow-growing tumours. To date, there are already many trials showing promising results of ion beam therapy in different oncological settings. For example, ion beam therapy in paediatric patients has reduced integral dose exposure, which in turn decreased late morbidity and has potentially reduced the risk of secondary cancer [23, 24]. In highly radioresistant tumours of the skull base, such as chordomas and chondrosarcomas, promising results could be achieved by the use of carbon ion radiotherapy, even in cases of re-irradiation [25]. Glioblastoma and pancreatic cancer, where radiotherapy is still very limited, could also be successfully treated by carbon ion radiotherapy [26–28]. However, it is still of utmost importance to evaluate the clinical opportunities of ion beam therapy, which is why its prognostic influence on the general outcome has to be further investigated in clinical trials and preclinical research.

In summary, we have witnessed tremendous advances in various fields of radiation oncology, which have contributed to the overall improved prognosis of cancer patients. These advances form the basis for current preclinical and clinical research, which will strengthen the positioning of radiation oncology as an essential pillar of oncological care.

Matthias Guckenberger, Zurich
Stephanie E. Combs, Munich
Daniel Zips, Tübingen

References

1 Allemani C, et al: Global surveillance of cancer survival 1995–2009: analysis of individual data for 25,676,887 patients from 279 population-based registries in 67 countries (CONCORD-2). Lancet 2015;385:977–1010.
2 Mitchell MJ, Jain RK, Langer R: Engineering and physical sciences in oncology: challenges and opportunities. Nat Rev Cancer 2017;17:659–675.
3 Baumann, M, et al: Radiation oncology in the era of precision medicine. Nat Rev Cancer 2016;16:234–249.
4 Rodemann HP, Datta NR, Bodis S: Molecular radiation biology/oncology and its impact on preclinical and clinical research in radiotherapy. Radiother Oncol 2017;124:339–343.
5 Kelderman S, Schumacher TN, Haanen JB: Acquired and intrinsic resistance in cancer immunotherapy. Mol Oncol 2014;8:1132–1139.
6 Van Limbergen EJ, et al: Combining radiotherapy with immunotherapy: the past, the present and the future. Br J Radiol 2017;90:20170157.
7 Kepka L, Socha J: PET-CT use and the occurrence of elective nodal failure in involved field radiotherapy for non-small cell lung cancer: a systematic review. Radiother Oncol 2015;115:151–156.
8 Rasch C, et al: Definition of the prostate in CT and MRI: a multi-observer study. Int J Radiat Oncol Biol Phys 1999;43:57–66.

9 Ling CC, et al: Towards multidimensional radiotherapy (MD-CRT): biological imaging and biological conformality. Int J Radiat Oncol Biol Phys 2000;47:551–560.
10 Lambin P, et al: Radiomics: the bridge between medical imaging and personalized medicine. Nat Rev Clin Oncol 2017;14:749–762.
11 Bogowicz M, et al: Post-radiochemotherapy PET radiomics in head and neck cancer – the influence of radiomics implementation on the reproducibility of local control tumor models. Radiother Oncol 2017;125:385–391.
12 Chun SG, et al: Impact of intensity-modulated radiation therapy technique for locally advanced non-small-cell lung cancer: a secondary analysis of the NRG Oncology RTOG 0617 Randomized Clinical Trial. J Clin Oncol 2017;35:56–62.
13 Sheets NC, et al: Intensity-modulated radiation therapy, proton therapy, or conformal radiation therapy and morbidity and disease control in localized prostate cancer. JAMA 2012;307:1611–1620.
14 Voet PW, et al: Toward fully automated multicriterial plan generation: a prospective clinical study. Int J Radiat Oncol Biol Phys 2013;85:866–872.
15 Schubert C, et al: Intercenter validation of a knowledge based model for automated planning of volumetric modulated arc therapy for prostate cancer. The experience of the German RapidPlan Consortium. PLoS One 2017;12:e0178034.

16 Acharya S, et al: Online magnetic resonance image guided adaptive radiation therapy: first clinical applications. Int J Radiat Oncol Biol Phys 2016;94:394–403.
17 Lax I, et al: Stereotactic radiotherapy of malignancies in the abdomen: methodological aspects. Acta Oncol 1994;33:677–683.
18 Vansteenkiste J, et al: Early and locally advanced non-small-cell lung cancer (NSCLC): ESMO clinical practice guidelines for diagnosis, treatment and follow-up. Ann Oncol 2013;24(suppl 6):vi89–vi98.
19 Chang JY, et al: Stereotactic ablative radiotherapy versus lobectomy for operable stage I non-small-cell lung cancer: a pooled analysis of two randomised trials. Lancet Oncol 2015;16:630–637.
20 Gomez DR, et al: Local consolidative therapy versus maintenance therapy or observation for patients with oligometastatic non-small-cell lung cancer without progression after first-line systemic therapy: a multicentre, randomised, controlled, phase 2 study. Lancet Oncol 2016;17:1672–1682.
21 Tanadini-Lang S, et al: Nomogram based overall survival prediction in stereotactic body radiotherapy for oligometastatic lung disease. Radiother Oncol 2017;123:182–188.
22 Kroeze SG, et al: Toxicity of concurrent stereotactic radiotherapy and targeted therapy or immunotherapy: a systematic review. Cancer Treat Rev 2017;53:25–37.

23 Meadows AT, et al: Second neoplasms in survivors of childhood cancer: findings from the Childhood Cancer Survivor Study cohort. J Clin Oncol 2009;27: 2356–2362.
24 Eaton BR, et al: Clinical outcomes among children with standard-risk medulloblastoma treated with proton and photon radiation therapy: a comparison of disease control and overall survival. Int J Radiat Oncol Biol Phys 2016;94: 133–138.
25 Uhl M, et al: Active raster scanning with carbon ions: reirradiation in patients with recurrent skull base chordomas and chondrosarcomas. Strahlenther Onkol 2014;190:686–691.
26 Shinoto M, et al: Carbon ion radiation therapy with concurrent gemcitabine for patients with locally advanced pancreatic cancer. Int J Radiat Oncol Biol Phys 2016;95:498–504.
27 Shinoto M, et al: Phase 1 trial of preoperative, short-course carbon-ion radiotherapy for patients with resectable pancreatic cancer. Cancer 2013;119:45–51.
28 Combs SE, et al: Comparison of carbon ion radiotherapy to photon radiation alone or in combination with temozolomide in patients with high-grade gliomas: explorative hypothesis-generating retrospective analysis. Radiother Oncol 2013;108:132–135.

Guckenberger M, Combs SE, Zips D (eds): Advances in Radiotherapy.
Prog Tumor Res. Basel, Karger, 2018, vol 44, pp 1–10 (DOI: 10.1159/000486981)

Principles and Developments in Cancer Immunotherapy and Approaches for Combination with Tumour Irradiation

Franziska Eckert · Stephan Huber

Department of Radiation Oncology, Eberhard Karls University of Tübingen, Tübingen, Germany

Abstract

Different immunotherapy concepts developed over recent decades include immune checkpoint inhibition, vaccination, and T cell-engaging therapies, as well as effectors on the immunosuppressive tumour microenvironment. For all these immunotherapy approaches, combination studies with tumour irradiation have been performed in vivo and in the clinic. The results point towards possible opportunities for combination therapies to improve patient outcome. © 2018 S. Karger AG, Basel

Historical Overview of Immunotherapy Development

Cancer Immunotherapy with Induced Erysipelas
Historically, one of the first systematic approaches to immunotherapy for cancer was therapy with induced erysipelas performed by William Coley [1]. Inoculation of bacteria (*Streptococcus pyogenes*) locally at the tumour site when followed by signs of local and systemic infection led to tumour shrinkage and in some patients to complete and lasting responses of inoperable cancers [2]. The mixture of heat-inactivated Streptococci and heat inactivated Serratia became known as "Coley's toxin" [3].

Immunological Features in the "Hallmarks of Cancer"
After having focused on the 3 main pillars of oncology (surgery, radiotherapy, and chemotherapy) and the development of targeted therapies, the oncological field came back to acknowledging the role of the immune system and the efficacy of immunotherapy only recently. Thus, Hanahan and Weinberg [4] added 2 immunological features of enabling capacity and emerging hallmark in their updated review on tumour biology in 2011, namely "tumour promoting inflammation" and "evading immune destruction." Compartments of the innate immune system, such as M2 polarised macrophages, especially contribute to cancer cell survival, angiogenesis, and invasion [5]. In addition, the release of reactive oxygen species by macrophages has a mutagenic effect which can

molecular patterns, or DAMPs, activating the innate immunity and thus paving the way for effective tumour eradication [52–55]. Surviving tumour cells show upregulation of MHC-I and NKG2D [56] and become more vulnerable to attack by T cells. In addition, the release of proinflammatory cytokines triggered by tissue damage through irradiation may polarise the immune response to a Th1 type, which also helps to support antitumour immunity. Primed and activated T cells will enter irradiated tumours more easily than nonirradiated tumours, for example due to increased expression of VCAM-1 in the tumour vasculature and the altered cytokine milieu [57, 58]. In in vivo models with more than 1 tumour in 1 animal, the combination of radiation and immunotherapy has been described to elicit "abscopal responses," with tumour shrinkage not only in the irradiated tumour but also in non-irradiated lesions in the same animal [59, 60]. This effect has also been observed in the clinic [61–63]. However, irradiation alone only rarely leads to antitumour immune effects in patients, and abscopal effects have only been described in a few case reports. This might be explained by the upregulation of immunosuppressive mechanisms, like the induction of Treg cells and a possible Th2 polarisation after irradiation [64, 65]. Tumours might also be able to upregulate PD-L1 after irradiation [66].

Combination Concepts

Combination of Irradiation and Immune Checkpoint Inhibition
As immune checkpoint inhibition is the most advanced modality for cancer immunotherapy, the combination with irradiation has been evaluated in a number of preclinical and clinical studies. CTLA-4 blockade showed enhanced local and distant control in combination with irradiation in in vivo models of breast cancer, colorectal cancer, and glioma [67–69]. Similar results have been reported for the combination of radiation with PD-1 blockade [70,

71]. However, the first clinical data showed only limited additive or synergistic activity of combination regimens compared to immune checkpoint inhibition alone in melanoma [72] and prostate cancer [73, 74]. The limited success might be due to the selection of patient cohorts, suboptimal radiation regimes, or problems in timing [75]. In vivo studies also suggest that triple combination of CTLA-4 blockade, PD-1 blockade, and radiation might be able to overcome resistance mechanisms [66]. Ongoing clinical trials in different cancer entities (for example CTLA-4 blockade, summarised by Vanpouille-Box et al. [75]) will show whether and how patients might benefit from combination therapies.

Antigen Release through Irradiation and Cancer Vaccines
The immunogenic cell death induced by irradiation can synergise with anticancer vaccines. The combination has been evaluated for dendritic cell vaccines, whole-tumour cell vaccines, and viral vaccines, as well as peptide and nucleic acid vaccines [76].

For virus-induced cancers, irradiation might be combined with vaccines targeting the respective virus. One example is HPV-associated head and neck cancer, where preclinical data have shown pronounced combination effects [77]. RNA-based vaccination in combination with irradiation has been evaluated for a Lewis Lung Cancer model and showed promising results [78], so that the concept has been translated into a clinical phase Ib trial [79]. A poxvirus-based vaccine was evaluated in combination with curative radiotherapy for prostate cancer [80]. However, the long-term follow-up did not show a significant difference to standard treatment concerning prostate-specific antigen control and immune responses [81].

T Cell Effects and T Cell-Engaging Therapy
One of the main immunological effects of irradiation is to facilitate T cell infiltration in tumours. Non-irradiated tumours often have a tumour-

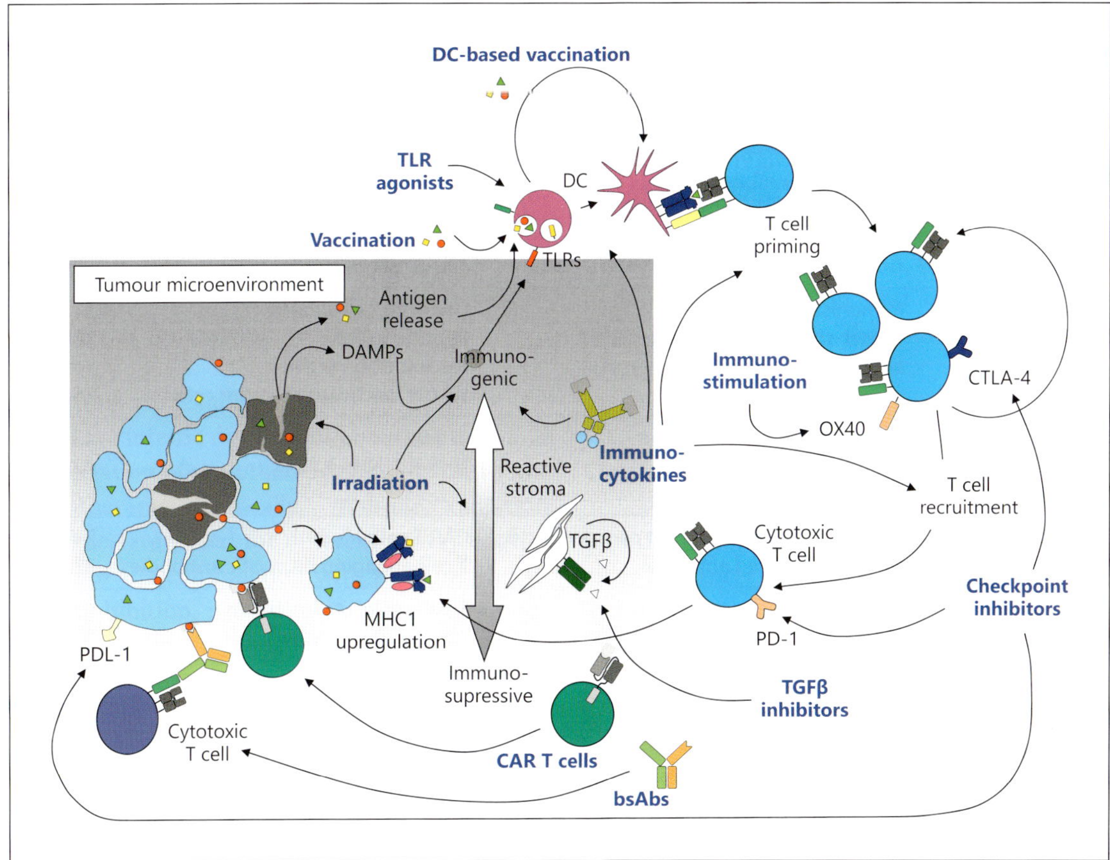

Fig. 1. Antitumour immune responses are dependent on neoantigen presentation by dendritic cells and dendritic cell activation leading to T cell activation and expansion. Tumour-targeting T cells have to enter the tumour and overcome the immunosuppressive tumour microenvironment. Different immunotherapeutic strategies alter this process at different stages and might be beneficial in combination with irradiation based on different conceptual ideas of interaction, as displayed.

suppressive microenvironment with the T cells present located at the borders of the tumour without being able to exert their antitumour function. Irradiation can change this picture and T cells will enter the tumours and begin to be activated [57, 58]. This is the rationale for combining irradiation with T cell-engaging therapies. Chimeric antigen receptor T cells as well as T cell-engaging bispecific antibodies are able to transform every intratumoural T cell into an antitumour T cell irrespective of their T cell receptor specificity [82–84] so that the combination with irradiation

might elicit additive or synergistic effects. Yet, the first preclinical data showed a dependency of response on initial tumour size with a negative effect of combination treatment on tumour control for some subgroups [85].

Tumour Microenvironment and Cytokine-Based Therapies

The tumour microenvironment engages different tumour-suppressive mechanisms, which might even be more pronounced after irradiation. Immunocytokines are able to overcome this

90 Schilbach K, et al: Cancer-targeted IL-12 controls human rhabdomyosarcoma by senescence induction and myogenic differentiation. Oncoimmunology 2015; 4:e1014760.

91 Paoloni M, et al: Defining the pharmacodynamic profile and therapeutic index of NHS-IL12 immunocytokine in dogs with malignant melanoma. PLoS One 2015;10:e0129954.

92 Eckert F, et al: Enhanced binding of necrosis-targeting immunocytokine NHS-IL12 after local tumour irradiation in murine xenograft models. Cancer Immunol Immunother 2016;65:1003–1013.

93 Kang J, Demaria S, Formenti S: Current clinical trials testing the combination of immunotherapy with radiotherapy. J Immunother Cancer 2016;4:51.

94 Kulzer L, et al: Norm- and hypo-fractionated radiotherapy is capable of activating human dendritic cells. J Immunotoxicol 2014;11:328–336.

95 Gandhi SJ, et al: Awakening the immune system with radiation: optimal dose and fractionation. Cancer Lett 2015;368: 185–190.

96 Golden EB, et al: An abscopal response to radiation and ipilimumab in a patient with metastatic non-small cell lung cancer. Cancer Immunol Res 2013;1:365–372.

97 Eckert F, Jelas I, Oehme M, Huber SM, Sonntag K, Welker C, Gillies SD, Strittmatter W, Zips D, Handgretinger R, Schilbach K: Tumor-targeted IL-12 combined with local irradiation leads to systemic tumor control via abscopal effects in vivo. Oncoimmunology 2017; 6:e1323161.

Franziska Eckert, MD
Department of Radiation Oncology, Eberhard Karls University of Tübingen
Hoppe-Seyler-Strasse 3
DE–72076 Tübingen (Germany)
E-Mail franziska.eckert@med.uni-tuebingen.de

Guckenberger M, Combs SE, Zips D (eds): Advances in Radiotherapy.
Prog Tumor Res. Basel, Karger, 2018, vol 44, pp 11–24 (DOI: 10.1159/000486985)

Imageable Biomarkers for Radiotherapy Response

W. Woliner-van der Weg · P.N. Span · P.M. Braam · J. Bussink

Department of Radiation Oncology, Radboud University Medical Center, Nijmegen, The Netherlands

Abstract

Ideally, each patient with a malignancy who is eligible for radiation therapy should receive the most tumoricidal form of this this treatment with the lowest possible risk of toxicity. To overcome radiotherapy resistance, some patients would benefit from a more aggressive approach. This could be treatment intensification, for example by acceleration of the treatment to prevent the negative effects of accelerated tumor cell proliferation, or by boosting certain areas to specifically address intrinsic radioresistance, or a combination of radiotherapy with, for example, a hypoxic cell sensitizer or chemotherapy to reduce the radiotherapy resistance caused by hypoxia. For some patients, one of these approaches can be beneficial but for others could lead to unacceptable side effects. Therefore, it is highly desirable to make the selection upfront. The use of imageable biomarkers could be the key to a more patient-tailored treatment. Different biomarkers for hypoxia and proliferation that could be valuable for radiotherapy are discussed here, including their mechanism, the imaging procedure, quantification, and the value of the results.

© 2018 S. Karger AG, Basel

In recent decades, technological developments in treatment planning and image-guided radiotherapy have led to increased precision of radiation treatments. To make the next big step, a more patient-customized treatment is anticipated, with radiation doses as high as needed for a tumoricidal effect, and as low as possible to minimize the risk of healthy tissue toxicity. To achieve this goal, the biological effectiveness can be improved for instance by treatment acceleration, i.e., reducing the overall treatment time, or by combining radiotherapy with a radiosensitizer. Selecting the most appropriate treatment for a patient requires knowledge about the potential effect of different types of treatment on an individual level. Individual biological information, obtained by the imaging of biomarkers, could be the key to move from population-based to patient-tailored treatments [1].

There is no clear definition of "biomarkers," but, in general, the term means "objective, quantifiable characteristics of a biological process that can be measured accurately and is reproducible"

[2]. We use the term biomarker for quantifiable biological characteristics that can predict treatment efficacy, and, although a broad range of biomarkers can be included, e.g., patient weight, or pulmonary function, we confine ourselves to noninvasively imageable biomarkers that give an indication with respect to the biology of the tumor microenvironment.

In contrast to biopsies and characteristics derived from blood samples, imaging provides 3-dimensional (3D) information about tumor characteristics. At the cost of a relatively low resolution – that is relative to the microscopic or even molecular level at which resistance takes place – information is obtained for the whole tumor. In general, imaging can be performed repetitively and, apart from the additional radiation burden or administration of contrast fluid or radioactive compounds, it is noninvasive. Another advantage of imaging is its already defined role in diagnosis and patient management [1].

Since the early 1980s, when computed tomography (CT) imaging became widely used, tumor size has been the best-known imaging biomarker. Volumetric measurements also remain the basis for the evaluation of tumor response according to the RECIST-criteria. However, size is a biomarker reflecting the final part of a biological response, i.e., for a size reduction tumor cells must have died and been removed from the tissue. Thus, it is a "late" marker, delaying evaluation up to 12 weeks following radiotherapy since the principle of cell kill resulting from radiotherapy is predominantly caused by mitotic catastrophe. Receptor expression, proliferation, metabolism, vascularization, diffusion, and perfusion change can be detected earlier than a difference in size [3] (Fig. 1a, b). Therefore, molecular and functional imaging are repeatedly suggested for early detection of treatment response, especially when targeted therapies are given, for instance in combination with radiotherapy [4–6]. Also, treatment modification to overcome radiation resistance, for instance modifying tumor cell hypoxia, may also be visualized at an earlier stage [7].

Many potential imaging biomarkers for the prediction of treatment response and treatment guidance have been described [8–12]. Before routine clinical use, these biomarkers have to bridge 2 "translational gaps": first to become a reliable tool for medical research, and then to become a reliable, practical tool for clinical decision making [13]. Of the many tracers suggested to have potential, only a few make it into routine clinical practice. In radiotherapy, CT imaging (with or without i.v. contrast, 3D or 4D) is routinely used for treatment planning and evaluation. Magnetic resonance imaging (MRI) is increasingly being applied for target definition and treatment evaluation. Positron emission tomography (PET) is mainly used with fluorodeoxyglucose (^{18}F-FDG), visualizing glucose metabolism as a surrogate for tumor activity, and used for diagnosis and tumor delineation. Mostly cone-beam CT or, to a lesser extent, albeit with a high potential, MRI is being applied for position verification.

Both PET and MRI can give more biological information than is currently obtained. Here, we focus on imaging biomarkers, mainly PET based, that can contribute to radiotherapy both for planning and evaluation purposes. These biomarkers should at least have the potential to allow the selection of patients benefiting from an adapted treatment (e.g., boost, hypofractionation, hypoxic cell sensitization) or exclude patients from radiotherapy that would not benefit because of radioresistance. Therefore, we will focus on 2 of the most important mechanisms of radioresistance: hypoxia and accelerated tumor cell proliferation [14] (Fig. 2).

For those who are not familiar with the technical aspects of PET, we begin by briefly explaining this technique. This is followed by the actual description of imaging hypoxia and proliferation biomarkers for radiotherapy – what do they exactly visualize and how can this be useful for radiotherapy?

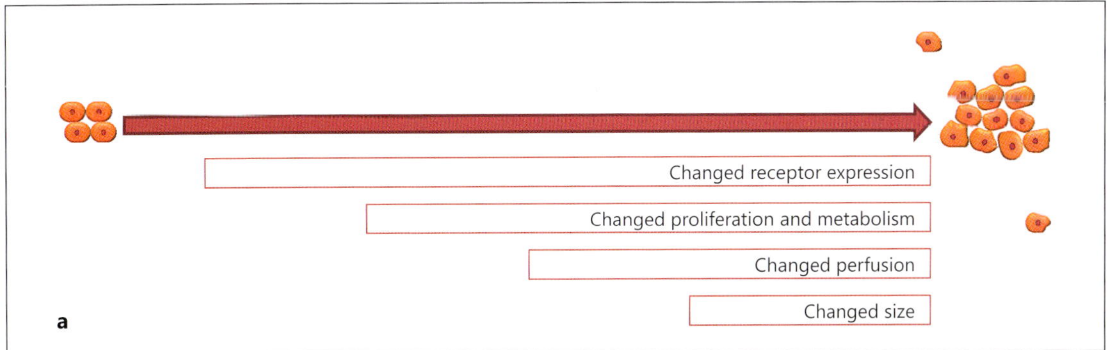

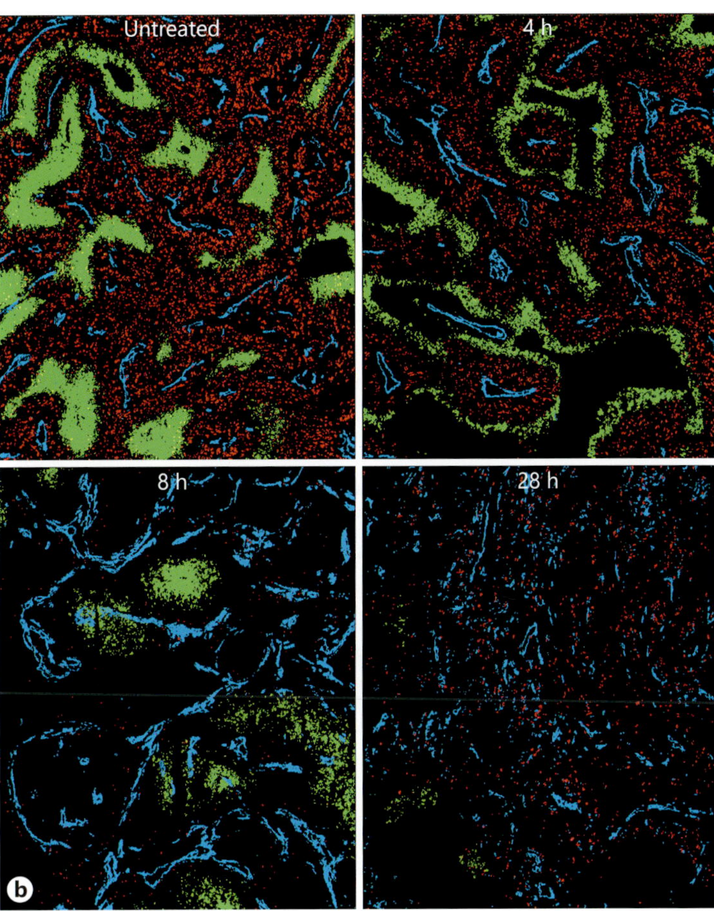

Fig. 1. a Before the change in size, other changes in tumor (cell) characteristics could be used to predict tumor development or the effect of radiotherapy. Since proliferation is an early biomarker, imaging of proliferation can be valuable for early response prediction or pretreatment patient selection. **b** Human tumor xenografted head and neck squamous cell carcinomas treated with a single dose of 10-Gy photons. Note the differences in rates of a changing microenvironment. Within 6–8 h a drastic reduction in hypoxia (pimonidazole, green) is observed lasting beyond the last time point at 28 h. The rate at which proliferation (BrdUrd, red) changes occur is faster and shorter; recovery of tumor cell proliferation can already be observed at 28 h. Blood vessels are blue (9F1). (Previously published by Bussink et al. [56].)

PET Imaging

PET imaging relies on the emission of a positron. Within a few millimeters of maximal emission, this (positive) positron undergoes annihilation with a (negative) electron, converting the masses into one pair of so-called annihilation photons. These 511-keV photons are emitted in about 180° opposing directions ("back-to-back"). The photons are almost simultaneously (within 6–12

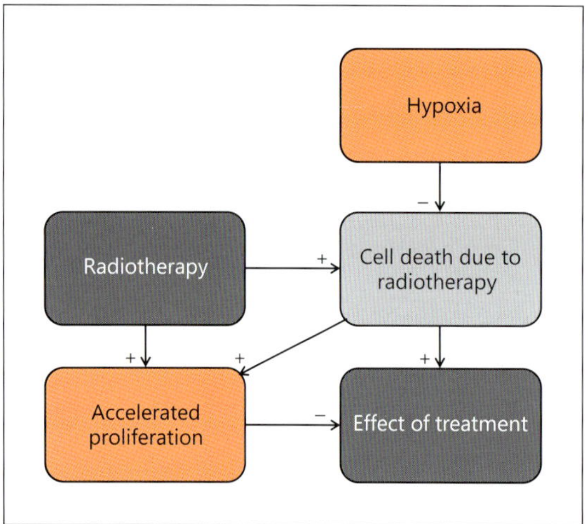

Fig. 2. The influence of hypoxia and accelerated proliferation on the effect of radiotherapy.

ns) detected by the PET, which allows assignment of the photons to annihilation on a certain "line of response." PET typically has an image resolution of about 5 mm, which is much larger than the scale of the biological processes being visualized.

Within human tissue, the half-value layer of 511-keV photons is about 7 cm. Therefore, PET images need to be corrected for attenuation. Commonly, a low-dose CT is made consecutively and used for attenuation correction. This CT is also the anatomical reference image for the PET images, to aid interpretation. Depending on the investigated tissue, it is important to understand that CT usually leads to a "snapshot" image, while PET acquisition takes at least minutes and, without a gating image, is influenced by breathing motion and heart-beating, etc. This can lead to a local mismatch between PET and CT.

PET imaging can be performed with different radionuclides, as long as positrons are being emitted. The radionuclide can be attached to a "tracer," which is used as a vehicle and key, to lead the radionuclide to and into the tissue to be visualized. After intravenous administration, uptake and accumulation of the tracer in the target tissue takes some time. For ^{18}F-FDG PET this is about 1 h. For hypoxia imaging this can rise up to 4 h. If not enough time is allowed every tracer is reduced to a marker of blood perfusion. Therefore, the half-life of the radionuclide should be long enough for sufficient signal at the moment of imaging. To limit the radiation dose due to the administration, the half-life should not be unnecessary long. The most used radionuclide is ^{18}F, which has a half-life of 110 min. ^{18}F needs to be produced in a cyclotron, but due to this half-life it can be transported after production and be used at a different location. It does not need to be produced and used on site.

The resulting PET images are quantitative, which means that voxel values correspond to the actual activity in the patient (Bq/mL). Assessment of the uptake is usually done by calculation of the "standard uptake value" (SUV) or a derivative. The SUV is the uptake in the tissue, corrected for injected activity and patient weight. In other words, if the activity was completely homogeneously distributed over the entire body, the SUV would be 1 in the whole body. If it all accumulated in half the body, the SUV would be 2 in that part and 0 in the remainder. Frequently used derivatives are SUVmax (maximum SUV in the region of interest; ROI), SUVmean (average SUV in the ROI), SUVpeak (the average SUV of a 2D or 3D ROI with a 1.2-cm diameter over the tumor area with the highest uptake [15]), MTV (metabolic tumor volume, tumor volume measured with a fixed or relative threshold, e.g., 50% of the max [15]), and TLG (total lesion glycolysis = MTV × SUVmean).

In the case of very local uptake (<2× full width of half the maximum of the system), the partial volume effect should be considered. Spillover in neighboring voxels reduces the visualized activity, and therefore reduces the SUV.

Since there are so many options in preparation, image acquisition, and image interpretation,

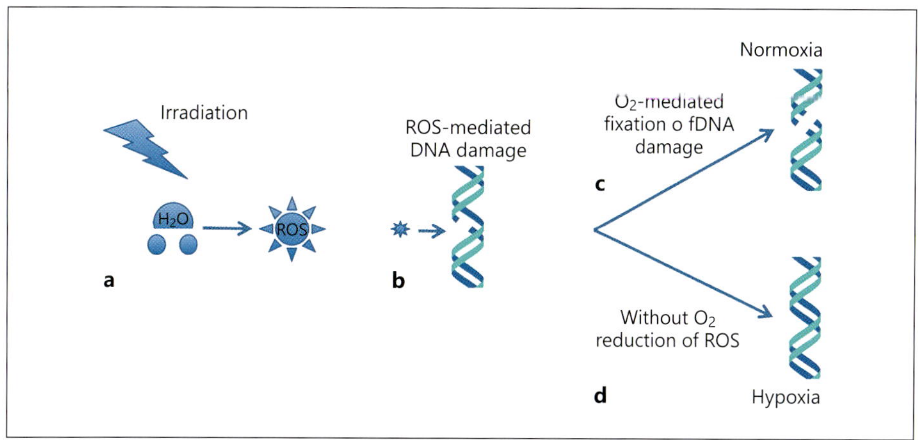

Fig. 3. Why oxygen is a radiosensitizer: the oxygen fixation theory. **a** Irradiation with high energy photons or electrons generates reactive oxygen species (ROS). **b** ROS mediates DNA damage. **c** Under normoxia, O2 mediates the fixation of this damage, leading to detrimental double strand DNA breaks, whereas (**d**) under hypoxia, the ROS is reduced.

standardization is required to enable comparison and combination of clinical study results. Therefore, the availability of guidelines of the European Association of Nuclear Medicine (EANM) [15] and their EARL accreditation program, used for the harmonization of acquisition and interpretation within multicenter trials, are also valuable in view of biomarker research.

In general, it should be kept in mind that the PET voxel size does not match with the microscopic level on which the biological processes occur that we are interested in [16]. This complicates the identification of small-scale heterogeneity in uptake. Nevertheless, considering this and being aware of what is actually measured and the robustness of the measurement, there are PET-based imaging biomarkers that are worth further investigation.

Imageable Biomarkers

Imaging of Hypoxia
One of the most interesting imageable biomarkers related to radioresistance is hypoxia, i.e., the lack of oxygen often encountered in solid tumors. Hypoxia is generally referred to as the status when the oxygen level in tissues is below physiological levels. Radiobiological hypoxia usually refers to the very low levels that are required to make cells maximally radioresistant, which is at levels less than 5–10 mm Hg [17]. Hypoxic cells are up to 3 times more radioresistant than normoxic cells, and hypoxia is associated with (radio)therapy resistance and poor prognosis [18]. Therefore, imaging of hypoxia in tumors can be useful in establishing a prognosis, might predict response to (radiation) treatment, and can be used to personalize cancer treatment.

Hypoxia and Radioresistance
Several mechanisms can explain the lack of radiosensitivity in hypoxic tumors. Firstly, the effect of DNA damage induced by radiotherapy depends on the presence of oxygen. While DNA damage induced by free radicals can be restored in hypoxic areas, in the presence of oxygen the damage becomes permanent and irreparable. In other words, oxygen fixates the damage, and therefore

this mechanism is called the oxygen fixation hypothesis (Fig. 3). The oxygen fixation hypothesis contributes to the so-called oxygen enhancement ratio (OER), which indicates that cells are 2–3 times more radiosensitive in the presence of oxygen relative to the absence of oxygen. The maximum of the OER curve lies at pO_2 >10–15 mm Hg, above which the radiosensitivity does not increase much further. At a pO_2 of about 2–5 mm Hg, the OER is reduced to about half the maximum level [19].

Secondly, tumor cells adopt a number of programs to survive a detrimental hypoxic microenvironment, which include hypoxia-inducible factor (HIF)-induced gene expression, the unfolded protein response (UPR) and – thereby among others – autophagy and mammalian targeting of rapamycin (mTOR) [20]. These programs are all directed to the survival of (tumor) cells under metabolic stress and lead to apoptosis resistance, increased metastasis, and increased genomic stability, etc. Additionally, the HIF-1 regulation of glycolysis and the pentose phosphate pathway lead to an aberrant cellular metabolism that increases the antioxidant capacity of tumors, thereby countering the oxidative stress caused by irradiation [21]. Finally, hypoxia will also lead to selection of particular tumor clones that are resistant to hypoxia-induced cell death. Combined with increased genomic imbalance, hypoxia will thus lead to the selection of more aggressive subclones, harboring p53 mutations, for example [22].

Causes of Hypoxia
The blood supply of a malignant tumor is often suboptimal as the vascular network is immature and chaotic. This chaotic vascular network results in tumor hypoxia [23]. Mainly 2 forms of hypoxia exist [14]: chronic, diffusion-limited and acute perfusion-limited hypoxia [17]. In chronic hypoxia, tumor cells at a certain distance from blood vessels (100–150 μm) are beyond the maximal diffusion distance for oxygen [14]. This distance is even shorter due to the increased oxygen consumption in rapidly dividing tumor cells, with chronic hypoxia depending on both supply and demand. (Chronically) hypoxic tumor cells have exceeded the oxygen capacity of the newly formed vascular network. This is due to the fact that the new microvasculature is often insufficient in providing normoxic circumstances in the distant tumor areas and will thereby contribute to diffusion-limited hypoxia [23]. Anemia and hypoxemia can also cause, and certainly contribute to, chronic hypoxia [17]. Imaging tracers are predominantly markers for chronic hypoxia, because hypoxia needs to persist for a period of time that is sufficiently long enough to allow targeting and binding [14].

Another form of hypoxia is acute, perfusion-limited hypoxia, which is caused by the transient opening and closing of blood vessels, producing fluctuations in perfusion of tumor regions, and changes in oxygen tension [14]. The structural and functional abnormalities in the newly formed vasculature cause malfunctioning of the blood supply. This in turn results in an unstable blood flow causing intermittent hypoxia close to poorly organized vessels. This form of hypoxia is characterized by rapidly changing oxygen concentrations [23]. Acute hypoxia cannot be reliably imaged using tracers. Its relevance for prognosis is unclear, whereas (acute) hypoxia during radiation treatment will surely attenuate treatment efficacy. The chaotic and complex vascularization of tumors results in a mixture of areas of predominant acute, chronic, or a mixture of these 2 states of hypoxia.

Counteracting Hypoxia
When imaging is found to indicate a more hypoxic tumor, or establishes which parts of a solid tumor are more hypoxic than other parts, treatment can be personalized by dose modification or "dose painting." However, hypoxia might be an (additional) target for treatment itself, or may also be countered before or during radiotherapy

(hypoxia modification). Hypoxic cells within tumors can be targeted through so-called hypoxia sensitization using bioreductive compounds [24, 25]. Modification imaging of hypoxia could be essential, as hypoxia modification for less hypoxic tumors is not only a futile effort, but might even potentially harm the patient as treatment-related toxicity could increase with hypoxia-targeted therapy [23]. Several different approaches have been used to resensitize hypoxic tumors, especially in anemic patients, such as hyperbaric oxygen treatment, erythropoietin, or red blood cell transfusions. These have been largely unsuccessful, or even counterproductive [26, 27]. A successful hypoxia modification strategy is the breathing of carbogen in combination with nicotinamide, which in combination with accelerated radiotherapy (ARCON) led to an improved regional control in laryngeal cancer patients with hypoxic tumors [28], and particularly in anemic patients [29]. Another successful approach is combining radiotherapy with the oxygen-mimetic nimorazole, which selectively sensitizes hypoxic cells to ionizing radiation by replacing oxygen in the chemical reactions that lead to the production of DNA damage [30]. Imaging patients for a priori selection of hypoxic tumors will be of the utmost importance of determining the effect of hypoxia-modification strategies.

PET-Based Hypoxia Imaging
There are 2 main tracer classes for imaging of hypoxia, the ^{18}F-labeled nitroimidazole-like compounds and the Cu-labelled diacetyl-bis(N4-methylthiosemicarbazone) analogues (Cu-ATSM) [10]. Since ^{18}F-FDG-PET visualizes both aerobic and anaerobic glucose consumption, this tracer is not suited for visualization of the oxygenation status of tissue [14, 31].

Mechanism of Nitroimidazole Uptake in Hypoxic Tissue
After injection into the bloodstream of the patient, the radiolabeled nitroimidazole derivatives spread throughout the whole blood volume. The lipophilic nature of the compound leads to passive diffusion into cells [32]. Within the cells nitroimidazoles combine with an electron, which has a high affinity for nitroimidazole, especially the $-NO_2$ part. The electron and nitroimidazole form a radical anion: $-NO_2^-$. Although electrons have a high affinity for nitroimidazole, they have an even higher affinity for oxygen. In the presence of oxygen, the electron in the radical anion can be taken over by the oxygen and the nitroimidazole returns to its parent state and can exit the cell again [33]. In the case of hypoxia (pO_2 <10 mm Hg), binding to an electron is not irreversible and the reduction continues. The reduction product remains trapped in the cell. Reduction of nitroimidazoles relies on the presence of active tissue reductases, which means that only viable hypoxic cells accumulate the reduction products and apoptotic or necrotic cells do not [23]. The accumulation of reduction products in hypoxic cells is inversely proportional to the local pO_2 [10]. When nitroimidazoles are radiolabeled, the radioactivity also accumulates in the hypoxic cell, which enables visualization and quantification of vital tissue hypoxia by PET imaging.

Different Nitroimidazole-Based PET-Tracers
Of the different nitroimidazole-based PET-tracers, ^{18}F-fluoromisonidazole (^{18}F-FMISO) was the first and still remains the most extensively studied [32, 33]. Although there is only limited clinical experience with ^{18}F-FMISO, there are some useful reviews describing the proven, assumed, or hypothesized differences between different nitroimidazole-based tracers [10, 23, 32]. In validation studies, a good correlation between ^{18}F-FMISO, visualized by autoradiography, and immunohistochemical visualization of 2-nitroimidazole derivatives was found [34]. Furthermore, preclinical work showed that changes in hypoxia could, to a certain extent, and based on tissue architecture, be visualized and quantified with this compound [35].

^{18}F-FMISO has the limitation of slow pharmacokinetics (about 2 h minimum between administration and imaging) and a poor hypoxic versus normoxic tissue contrast (20–40% difference in uptake). Therefore, other nitroimidazole-based tracers were developed in order to overcome these shortcomings. The different nitroimidazole-based tracers show (small) differences in uptake and imaging characteristics. In general, compounds that are more hydrophilic have a higher clearance and therefore higher tumor-to-blood ratio (T/B) [23]. Overall, theoretical benefits of other tracers, as compared to ^{18}F-FMISO, only lead to relatively small advantages in clinical practice. ^{18}F- fluoroazomycinarabinofuranoside (^{18}F-FAZA) is one of the second-generation nitroimidazole compounds and, due to its reduced lipophilicity, it has a faster washout of normoxic tissue, leading to a higher tissue-to-muscle ratio (about 2.0 at 2 h postinjection) [32]. ^{18}F-HX4 is one of the other more hydrophilic tracers with a faster clearance than ^{18}F-FMISO. Other examples of nitroimidazole-based tracers are ^{18}F-EF3 and ^{18}F-EF5, which have a more complex but also more stable labeling chemistry. Unfortunately, in practice the potential advantage over ^{18}F-FMISO turned out to be limited [32].

Today, many different nitroimidazole-based tracers are under investigation and, while they all have a slightly different profile, it is difficult to predict which one has the best overall potential to succeed ^{18}F-FMISO as the leading hypoxia PET tracer.

In preclinical studies, tracers labeled with other positron-emitting radionuclides have also been tested. For example, ^{68}Ga has the advantage that it can easily be produced with a ^{68}Ge-^{68}Ga generator, which makes the imaging independent of the availability of a cyclotron. The disadvantage of ^{68}Ga is the shorter half-life compared to ^{18}F (68 min vs. 110 min), while uptake of the nitroimidazole-based tracers takes hours. These differently labeled tracers have not (yet) proved to be advantageous over ^{18}F-FMISO.

Imaging of Nitroimidazole-Based Tracers

In general, PET imaging is performed 2–4 h after the administration of the ^{18}F-labeled nitroimidazole-based tracer [33]. This period between administration and imaging is required for sufficient uptake and accumulation of the tracer in the hypoxic tissue. With ^{18}F having a half-life of 110 min, the signal increase due to higher levels of the tracer in hypoxic tissue is partly counteracted by the decay leading to rapid lowering of the PET signal. The detected signal is also influenced by blood perfusion, the distance of passive diffusion, and the image acquisition protocol. Hypoxic tumors are often hypoperfused, which can lead to underestimation of the hypoxia based on imaging of the tracer uptake [10], while imaging within a short interval after administration leads to overestimation from perfusion artifacts in a well-perfused tumor.

Ideally, a parameter representing the pO$_2$ would be calculated from the acquired data. Unfortunately, this is methodologically challenging due to the abovementioned confounders. Therefore, in general the SUV, T/B, and tumor-to-muscle ratios (T/M) are applied for analysis. Alternatively, the hypoxic volume and the hypoxic fraction can be used as parameters for the quantification of hypoxia [36]. The hypoxic fraction is the hypoxic volume, defined as the tumor volume with T/B or T/M above a certain threshold (e.g., >1.2 to >1.4 for ^{18}F-FMISO [32, 37]), divided by the total tumor volume. Some groups use more demanding pharmacokinetic modeling methods to improve quantification by maximal correction for perfusion; however, this is a procedure where the total imaging time is substantially longer, which is cumbersome for patients [38]. Apart from the SUV, these are all relative parameters and sensitive for "inter-corporal" properties (blood volume, perfusion, clearance rate), relying on the definition of representative reference volumes (blood or muscle). Also, the parameters may vary among different protocols (e.g., amount of tracer injected, reconstruction method, correction for breathing motion). Furthermore, the time after administration influences the values, since at later time points the blood will be further cleared, while the uptake in hypoxic tissue increases as long as there is supply of the tracer.

Since hypoxia is in general defined by a signal increase of only 20–40%, the signal-to-noise ratio needs to be maximal, especially for the detection of small hypoxic subvolumes. Besides taking advantage of the optimal imaging timeframe according to the clearance and decay, image noise can be reduced by increasing the acquisition time or the administered activity. The first is at the cost of time and patient discomfort, while the second is at the cost of a higher imaging-induced radiation dose. Compared to often-used ^{18}F-FDG-PET imaging protocols, the time per bed position is much longer. While ^{18}F-FDG-PET is frequently used as a whole body imaging method (e.g., 6 bed positions), tumor hypoxia imaging can mostly be limited to 1 or 2 bed positions only, which reduces the overall time required for imaging.

Mechanism of Cu-ATSM Uptake in Hypoxic Tissue

The other group of PET-based hypoxia tracers consists of Cu-ATSM compounds. Although the uptake mechanism of these tracers is not fully understood, it is known that the lipophilic molecule diffuses through the cell membrane, and within the cell the copper compound undergoes reduction by thiols: Cu(II)-ATSM is converted to Cu(I)-ATSM. In the case of hypoxia, this unstable complex undergoes further reduction and the resulting free Cu(I) becomes rapidly entrapped in intracellular proteins [32].

Experiences with Cu-ATSM

Experiences with Cu-ATSM vary between promising and disappointing. The advantage of Cu-ATSM compared to nitroimidazole compounds is the higher uptake in target tissue (T/M 3.0) within only 10–15 min [32]. However, there are doubts on the hypoxic selectivity since the Cu-ATSM uptake does not always correspond to the distribution of immunohistochemical markers, especially at early imaging timepoints (<16 h after injection) [39, 40]. In future it will be elucidated whether further development of Cu-ATSM tracers can overcome these doubts [10].

Advantages and Disadvantages of PET-Based Hypoxia Imaging

Besides being a time-consuming procedure with hours between administration and imaging and a poor contrast between hypoxic and normoxic tissue, PET-based hypoxia imaging has the major disadvantage of a low resolution, resulting in problematic detection of small but potentially relevant volumes of hypoxic tissue [23]. A more general challenge of hypoxia imaging is its dynamic nature; it remains questionable whether a single PET can provide enough reliable information to make the treatment dependent on this biomarker [41–43]. The advantage of imaging biomarkers for hypoxia is that they provide 3D information about the tumor tissue, in a noninvasive manner. This enables longitudinal monitoring and facilitates further research in this field.

MRI-Based Hypoxia Imaging

Besides PET, hypoxia and perfusion may also be visualized with MRI. Different MRI protocols have been suggested for this, for instance dynamic contrast enhanced (DCE) MRI in which gadolinium is typically used as a paramagnetic contrast agent. With DCE MRI, different parameters can be retrieved (e.g., k^{trans}/k_{ep}, v_e) for the visualization of tissue perfusion.

Reduced perfusion might indicate tumor hypoxia, and therefore DCE MRI can be used as a surrogate for hypoxia imaging. However, increased vascular permeability leads to higher intratumoral contrast agent levels, while it may be associated with increased hypoxia [37, 44].

Other examples of interesting sequences/ protocols, although not (yet) with a proven predictive value, are blood-oxygen level-dependent (BOLD) MRI [45], which visualizes the ratio between paramagnetic deoxyhemoglobin and diamagnetic oxyhemoglobin, and the less mature tissue oxygen level dependent (TOLD) MRI, and mapping of oxygen by imaging lipid relaxation enhancement (MOBILE). These could be used for the visualization of tissue oxygenation in water and in lipids, respectively [44].

In MRI, the acquisition itself can be performed with many different settings, and many different parameters can be retrieved from the acquired data. Without denying the value of this field of research, in depth discussion about the advantages and disadvantages of these different techniques and applications is not included here.

Imaging of Proliferation

Proliferation and Radioresistance

In cancer tissue, a typical misbalance between the rate of cell death and the rate of cell proliferation occurs, resulting in tumor growth. Generally, within tumor categories the tumors with the highest proliferation rate have (without treatment) the worst prognosis [12], although conflicting study results have been published [46]. Generally, a higher proliferation rate before treatment and early during treatment may be related to a worse response to radiotherapy [8, 16], and especially accelerated proliferation during the course of radiotherapy is related to a poorer outcome.

Causes of Accelerated Proliferation

Irradiation results in the killing of well-oxygenated tumor cells, and therefore the tumor volume reduces. For the remaining malignant cells this leads to improved supply of oxygen and nutrition, a process referred to as "reoxygenation." Before therapy, these cells had to compete with many more tumor cells, which apparently would have led to spontaneous cell loss. Instead, due to radiotherapy, these cells are enabled for further proliferation. Proliferation itself is also stimulated in response to ionizing radiation [47]. This mechanism of proliferation of tumor cells, stimulated or enabled by radiotherapy, is called accelerated repopulation [48].

Counteracting Radioresistance due to Proliferation

Especially in fast-responding tumors, accelerated repopulation should be considered in the treatment design. Practically, specifically for head-and-neck squamous cell, and non-small-cell and small-cell lung cancer, this risk of repopulation during the treatment course is known [48]. In case of a longer treatment time, in these cancers accelerated repopulation plays a more prominent role and reduces the effectiveness of the radiotherapy. In this situation, tumor cell kill due to radiotherapy is attenuated by accelerated repopulation. In order to increase the treatment response by limiting the effect of accelerated repopulation, different approaches, such as accelerated radiotherapy or radiotherapy combined with another therapy, e.g., cetuximab, have been suggested. Since these are all at the cost of increased side effects [16], careful patient selection for this treatment modification is crucial. Imaging of proliferation, or accelerated repopulation, has the potency to select those patients or patient groups that require an intensified treatment, and could thereby contribute to an improved treatment outcome.

PET-Based Proliferation Imaging

One way to measure proliferation, or the effect of proliferation, is to measure the anatomical size of a tumor. Besides the delay in the visibility of the size-effect, even after weeks, size does not provide information on the tissue viability and is therefore an impaired biomarker. This makes ^{18}F-fluorothymidine (^{18}F-FLT) PET imaging, which visualizes cell proliferation, an attractive alternative. As it is not (yet) routinely used in the clinical practice of radiotherapy, it is an often-used imaging biomarker in research. Dose escalation based on ^{18}F-FLT PET has been suggested and was shown to be technically feasible [49].

Mechanism of ^{18}F-FLT Uptake and Accumulation

^{18}F-FLT is a radiolabeled variant of the nucleoside thymidine. After intravenous administration, ^{18}F-FLT gets transported into the cell by nucleoside transporters. The enzyme thymidine kinase 1 (TK1) leads to monophosphorylation of ^{18}F-FLT and thereby to trapping of ^{18}F-FLT in the cell [9, 31]. During the S-phase of the cell cycle (DNA synthesis) TK1 is increased about 10-fold [49], which makes ^{18}F-FLT visualize cell proliferation. This is confirmed by comparison of the ^{18}F-FLT uptake with the cellular proliferation biomarker Ki-67. Ki-67 is exclusively present in the active phases of the cell cycle, and therefore strictly associated with cell proliferation [50]. ^{18}F-FLT uptake and immunohistological analysis of Ki-67 expression showed a positive correlation [3], with the advantage of ^{18}F-FLT being noninvasive and providing information of the entire imaged volume (whole body is possible), at the cost of a much lower resolution.

Imaging of ^{18}F-FLT

^{18}F-FLT PET provides reproducible quantitative imaging results [3, 14]. A decrease in uptake of 20–25% is greater than the reproducibility error [31] and can therefore be attributed to a decrease in proliferation. Imaging can be performed about 1 h after administration of the ^{18}F-FLT, which is similar to the incubation period for imaging of ^{18}F-FDG, the frequently used glucose analogue for PET imaging. Beyond 1 h of incubation, proliferation might be underestimated by leakage of the metabolite back into the blood [51].

Compared to FDG, FLT has a lower tumor uptake. For example, for contouring of the functional tumor volume, for FLT a threshold of 1.4 of the SUV results in a volume that is similar to the volume calculated with FDG with a 2.5 threshold [52]. When using imaging of proliferation for early response prediction, it should be considered that, although proliferation is a characteristic of the tumor, it is not exclusively a tumor cell characteristic. Not only do proliferating tumor cells accumulate ^{18}F-FLT, but also, for example, proliferating B-lymphocytes in inflammatory lymph nodes [31] and in bone marrow [53]. Radiotherapy could increase uptake by inducing the proliferation of inflammatory cells in certain areas [31]. A relatively high background uptake in the liver and genitourinary system complicates the imaging of proliferation with ^{18}F-FLT in these areas. This limits the specificity of this biomarker and makes ^{18}F-FLT imaging better suited for the monitoring of treatment response than for staging [9, 14, 53].

For early response assessment, in head and neck cancer it was shown that already in the second week of treatment the decrease in ^{18}F-FLT uptake is indicative of the treatment outcome [54]. This allows the treatment protocol to be changed, for example accelerated. Since the ^{18}F-FLT uptake decreases at least during the first 4 weeks of therapy [31], the timing influences the outcome of the quantification.

The preparation of ^{18}F-FLT is different from ^{18}F-FDG. It requires, for example, a purification because of toxic side products. In contrast to the widely used FDG, in most institutes FLT is not easily available, which limits its use.

Perspective

Although ^{18}F-FLT-PET proved to assess radiotherapy treatment response earlier than ^{18}F-FDG-PET and CT tumor response [55], currently ^{18}F-FLT-PET is only applied within clinical studies.

Unfortunately, these studies are mostly single-center studies with a small sample size. Similar to studies applying ^{18}F-FDG-PET, standardization of ^{18}F-FLT-PET is required to enable the comparison and combination of clinical study results. Guidelines like the EANM guideline for ^{18}F-FDG-PET should also become available for other tracers, such as ^{18}F-FLT. This would stimulate harmonization and therefore increase the chance of success for these biomarkers.

The Future of Biomarker Imaging for Radiotherapy

Both hypoxia and the proliferation of imaging are illustrative for a more general challenge we face in the development of biomarker imaging for radiotherapy. Despite the many initiatives, based on many different biological characteristics, currently only a few biomarkers have the potency to enter clinical routine. These have to first overcome the challenge of nonuniformity in study designs, imaging, and quantification, which slows down further development by hampering the combination and comparison of results.

The value of the use of biomarkers lies in patient selection. The challenge of biomarker studies is to first select those patients that can demonstrate the working of the biomarker. By both biological and technical harmonization, biomarkers will further demonstrate their usefulness for radiotherapy. Biomarkers have the potency to be useful for both research and individual patients.

References

1 West CM, Huddart RA: Biomarkers and imaging for precision radiotherapy. Clin Oncol 2015;27:545–546.

2 Strimbu K, Tavel JA: What are biomarkers? Current Opin HIV AIDS 2010;5:463–466.

3 Weller A, O'Brien ME, Ahmed M, Popat S, Bhosle J, McDonald F, et al: Mechanism and non-mechanism based imaging biomarkers for assessing biological response to treatment in non-small cell lung cancer. Eur J Cancer 2016;59:65–78.

4 Desar IM, van Herpen CM, van Laarhoven HW, Barentsz JO, Oyen WJ, van der Graaf WT: Beyond RECIST: molecular and functional imaging techniques for evaluation of response to targeted therapy. Cancer Treat Rev 2009;35:309–321.

5 Serkova NJ, Eckhardt SG: Metabolic imaging to assess treatment response to cytotoxic and cytostatic agents. Front Oncol 2016;6:152.

6 Usmanij EA, de Geus-Oei LF, Troost EG, Peters-Bax L, van der Heijden EH, Kaanders JH, et al: ^{18}F-FDG PET early response evaluation of locally advanced non-small cell lung cancer treated with concomitant chemoradiotherapy. J Nucl Med 2013;54:1528–1534.

7 Grootjans W, de Geus-Oei LF, Troost EG, Visser EP, Oyen WJ, Bussink J: PET in the management of locally advanced and metastatic NSCLC. Nat Rev Clin Oncol 2015;12:395–407.

8 Prestwich RJ, Vaidyanathan S, Scarsbrook AF: Functional imaging biomarkers: potential to guide an individualised approach to radiotherapy. Clin Oncol 2015;27:588–600.

9 Croteau E, Renaud JM, Richard MA, Ruddy TD, Benard F, deKemp RA: PET metabolic biomarkers for cancer. Biomark Cancer 2016;8(suppl 2):61–69.

10 Fleming IN, Manavaki R, Blower PJ, West C, Williams KJ, Harris AL, et al: Imaging tumour hypoxia with positron emission tomography. Br J Cancer 2015;112:238–250.

11 Laking G, Price P: Radionuclide imaging of perfusion and hypoxia. Eur J Nucl Med Mol Imaging 2010;37(suppl 1):S20–S29.

12 Wahl RL, Herman JM, Ford E: The promise and pitfalls of positron emission tomography and single-photon emission computed tomography molecular imaging-guided radiation therapy. Semin Radiat Oncol 2011;21:88–100.

13 O'Connor JP, Aboagye EO, Adams JE, Aerts HJ, Barrington SF, Beer AJ, et al: Imaging biomarker roadmap for cancer studies. Nat Rev Clin Oncol 2017;14:169–186.

14 Bussink J, Kaanders JH, van der Graaf WT, Oyen WJ: PET-CT for radiotherapy treatment planning and response monitoring in solid tumors. Nat Rev Clin Oncol 2011;8:233–242.

15 Boellaard R, O'Doherty MJ, Weber WA, Mottaghy FM, Lonsdale MN, Stroobants SG, et al: FDG PET and PET/CT: EANM procedure guidelines for tumour PET imaging: version 1.0. Eur J Nucl Med Mol Imaging 2010;37:181–200.

16 Hoeben BA, Bussink J, Troost EG, Oyen WJ, Kaanders JH: Molecular PET imaging for biology-guided adaptive radiotherapy of head and neck cancer. Acta Oncol 2013;52:1257–1271.

17 Span PN, Bussink J: Biology of hypoxia. Semin Nucl Med 2015;45:101–109.

18 Horsman MR, Mortensen LS, Petersen JB, Busk M, Overgaard J: Imaging hypoxia to improve radiotherapy outcome. Nat Rev Clin Oncol 2012;9:674–687.

19 Padhani AR, Krohn KA, Lewis JS, Alber M: Imaging oxygenation of human tumours. Eur Radiol 2007;17:861–872.

20 Wouters BG, Koritzinsky M: Hypoxia signalling through mTOR and the unfolded protein response in cancer. Nat Rev Cancer 2008;8:851–864.

21 Meijer TW, Kaanders JH, Span PN, Bussink J: Targeting hypoxia, HIF-1, and tumor glucose metabolism to improve radiotherapy efficacy. Clin Cancer Res 2012;18:5585–5594.

22 Leszczynska KB, Foskolou IP, Abraham AG, Anbalagan S, Tellier C, Haider S, et al: Hypoxia-induced p53 modulates both apoptosis and radiosensitivity via AKT. J Clin Invest 2015;125:2385–2398.

23 Wijsman R, Kaanders JH, Oyen WJ, Bussink J: Hypoxia and tumor metabolism in radiation oncology: targets visualized by positron emission tomography. Q J Nucl Med Mol Imaging 2013;57:244–256.

24 Yaromina A, Krause M, Baumann M: Individualization of cancer treatment from radiotherapy perspective. Mol Oncol 2012;6:211–221.

25 Begg AC, Stewart FA, Vens C: Strategies to improve radiotherapy with targeted drugs. Nat Rev Cancer 2011;11:239–253.

26 Hoff CM, Lassen P, Eriksen JG, Hansen HS, Specht L, Overgaard M, et al: Does transfusion improve the outcome for HNSCC patients treated with radiotherapy? – Results from the randomized DAHANCA 5 and 7 trials. Acta Oncol 2011;50:1006–1014.

27 Lambin P, Ramaekers BL, van Mastrigt GA, et al: Erythropoietin as an adjuvant treatment with (chemo) radiation therapy for head and neck cancer. Cochrane Database Syst Rev 2009;3:CD006158.

28 Janssens GO, Rademakers SE, Terhaard CH, Doornaert PA, Bijl HP, van den Ende P, et al: Accelerated radiotherapy with carbogen and nicotinamide for laryngeal cancer: results of a phase III randomized trial. J Clin Oncol 2012;30:1777–1783.

29 Janssens GO, Rademakers SE, Terhaard CH, Doornaert PA, Bijl HP, van den Ende P, et al: Improved recurrence-free survival with ARCON for anemic patients with laryngeal cancer. Clin Cancer Res 2014;20:1345–1354.

30 Overgaard J, Hansen HS, Overgaard M, Bastholt L, Berthelsen A, Specht L, et al: A randomized double-blind phase III study of nimorazole as a hypoxic radiosensitizer of primary radiotherapy in supraglottic larynx and pharynx carcinoma. Results of the Danish Head and Neck Cancer Study (DAHANCA) Protocol 5-85. Radiother Oncol 1998;46:135–146.

31 Bussink J, van Herpen CM, Kaanders JH, Oyen WJ: PET-CT for response assessment and treatment adaptation in head and neck cancer. Lancet Oncol 2010;11:661–669.

32 Lopci E, Grassi I, Chiti A, Nanni C, Cicoria G, Toschi L, et al: PET radiopharmaceuticals for imaging of tumor hypoxia: a review of the evidence. Am J Nucl Med Mol Imaging 2014;4:365–384.

33 Krohn KA, Link JM, Mason RP: Molecular imaging of hypoxia. J Nucl Med 2008;49(suppl 2):129S–148S.

34 Troost EG, Laverman P, Philippens ME, Lok J, van der Kogel AJ, Oyen WJ, et al: Correlation of [^{18}F]FMISO autoradiography and pimonidazole (corrected) immunohistochemistry in human head and neck carcinoma xenografts. Eur J Nucl Med Mol Imaging 2008;35:1803–1811.

35 Troost EG, Bussink J, Kaanders JH, van Eerd J, Peters JP, Rijken PF, et al: Comparison of different methods of CAIX quantification in relation to hypoxia in three human head and neck tumor lines. Radiother Oncol 2005;76:194–199.

36 Shi K, Bayer C, Astner ST, Gaertner FC, Vaupel P, Schwaiger M, et al: Quantitative analysis of [^{18}F]FMISO PET for tumor hypoxia: correlation of modeling results with immunohistochemistry. Mol Imaging Biol 2017;19:120–129.

37 van Elmpt W, Zegers CM, Reymen B, Even AJ, Dingemans AM, Oellers M, et al: Multiparametric imaging of patient and tumour heterogeneity in non-small-cell lung cancer: quantification of tumour hypoxia, metabolism and perfusion. Eur J Nucl Med Mol Imaging 2016;43:240–248.

38 Taylor E, Yeung I, Keller H, Wouters BG, Milosevic M, Hedley DW, et al: Quantifying hypoxia in human cancers using static PET imaging. Phys Med Biol 2016;61:7957–7974.

39 Carlin S, Zhang H, Reese M, Ramos NN, Chen Q, Ricketts SA: A comparison of the imaging characteristics and microregional distribution of 4 hypoxia PET tracers. J Nucl Med 2014;55:515–521.

40 O'Donoghue JA, Zanzonico P, Pugachev A, Wen B, Smith-Jones P, Cai S, et al: Assessment of regional tumor hypoxia using ^{18}F-fluoromisonidazole and ^{64}Cu(II)-diacetyl-bis(N4-methylthiosemicarbazone) positron emission tomography: comparative study featuring microPET imaging, Po2 probe measurement, autoradiography, and fluorescent microscopy in the R3327-AT and FaDu rat tumor models. Int J Radiat Oncol Biol Phys 2005;61:1493–1502.

41 Ljungkvist AS, Bussink J, Kaanders JH, Rijken PF, Begg AC, Raleigh JA, et al: Hypoxic cell turnover in different solid tumor lines. Int J Radiat Oncol Biol Phys 2005;62:1157–1168.

42 Ljungkvist AS, Bussink J, Kaanders JH, van der Kogel AJ: Dynamics of tumor hypoxia measured with bioreductive hypoxic cell markers. Radiat Res 2007;167:127–145.

43 Ljungkvist AS, Bussink J, Rijken PF, Raleigh JA, Denekamp J, van der Kogel AJ: Changes in tumor hypoxia measured with a double hypoxic marker technique. Int J Radiat Oncol Biol Phys 2000;48:1529–1538.

44 Price JM, Robinson SP, Koh DM: Imaging hypoxia in tumours with advanced MRI. Q J Nucl Med Mol Imaging 2013;57:257–270.

45 King AD, Thoeny HC: Functional MRI for the prediction of treatment response in head and neck squamous cell carcinoma: potential and limitations. Cancer Imaging 2016;16:23.

46 Begg AC, Haustermans K, Hart AA, Dische S, Saunders M, Zackrisson B, et al: The value of pretreatment cell kinetic parameters as predictors for radiotherapy outcome in head and neck cancer: a multicenter analysis. Radiother Oncol 1999;50:13–23.

47 Perri F, Pacelli R, Della Vittoria Scarpati G, Cella L, Giuliano M, Caponigro F, et al: Radioresistance in head and neck squamous cell carcinoma: biological bases and therapeutic implications. Head Neck 2015;37:763–770.

48 Wang JZ, Li XA: Impact of tumor repopulation on radiotherapy planning. Int J Radiat Oncol Biol Phys 2005;61:220–227.

49 Troost EG, Bussink J, Hoffmann AL, Boerman OC, Oyen WJ, Kaanders JH: ^{18}F-FLT PET/CT for early response monitoring and dose escalation in oropharyngeal tumors. J Nucl Med 2010;51:866–874.

50 Scholzen T, Gerdes J: The Ki-67 protein: from the known and the unknown. J Cell Physiol 2000;182:311–322.

51 Soloviev D, Lewis D, Honess D, Aboagye E: [18F]FLT: an imaging biomarker of tumour proliferation for assessment of tumour response to treatment. Eur J Cancer 2012;48:416–424.

52 Debebe SA, Goryawala M, Adjouadi M, McGoron AJ, Gulec SA: ^{18}F-FLT positron emission tomography/computed tomography imaging in pancreatic cancer: determination of tumor proliferative activity and comparison with glycolytic activity as measured by ^{18}F-FDG positron emission tomography/computed tomography imaging. Mol Imaging Radionucl Ther 2016;25:32–38.

53 Tehrani OS, Shields AF: PET imaging of proliferation with pyrimidines. J Nucl Med 2013;54:903–912.

54 Hoeben BA, Troost EG, Span PN, van Herpen CM, Bussink J, Oyen WJ, et al: ^{18}F-FLT PET during radiotherapy or chemoradiotherapy in head and neck squamous cell carcinoma is an early predictor of outcome. J Nucl Med 2013;54:532–540.

55 Bollineni VR, Kramer GM, Jansma EP, Liu Y, Oyen WJ: A systematic review on [18F]FLT-PET uptake as a measure of treatment response in cancer patients. Eur J Cancer 2016;55:81–97.

56 Bussink J, Kaanders JH, Rijken PF, Raleigh JA, van der Kogel AJ: Changes in blood perfusion and hypoxia after irradiation of a human squamous cell carcinoma xenograft tumor line. Radiat Res 2000;153:398–404.

W. Woliner-van der Weg, PhD or J. Bussink, MD, PhD
Department of Radiation Oncology, Radboud University Medical Center
P.O. Box 9101
NL–6500 HB Nijmegen (115) (The Netherlands)
E-Mail wietske.woliner-vanderweg@radboudumc.nl or jan.bussink@radboudumc.nl

Guckenberger M, Combs SE, Zips D (eds): Advances in Radiotherapy.
Prog Tumor Res. Basel, Karger, 2018, vol 44, pp 25–40 (DOI: 10.1159/000486986)

Targeting Tumor Microenvironment and Metabolism to Overcome Radiation Resistance

Ashish Sharma · Martin Pruschy

Laboratory for Applied Radiobiology, Department of Radiation Oncology, University Hospital Zurich, University of Zurich, Zurich, Switzerland

Abstract

The tumor microenvironment comprises multiple different cell types and structural and functional components, and defines a unique tumor milieu on the individual tumor level. Several biological processes in the microenvironment are pivotal for tumor growth, like the formation of an intact tumor vasculature and the composition of the extracellular matrix. Furthermore, tumor heterogeneity also derives from the complex and dynamic interactions of the tumor cells with the stromal compartment during tumor growth and in response to treatment, and thereby represents a major treatment hurdle. Here we give an overview of the different entities of the tumor microenvironment and present their role in radiation resistance. Dynamic changes in response to irradiation will be outlined, and relevant approaches to target critical elements of the tumor microenvironment will be discussed. We are only now starting to understand how these different entities cooperate biologically, and thereby determine tumor aggressiveness and treatment resistance on the individual level. At the same time, these dynamic and even treatment-induced interactions within the tumor represent promising targets for novel combined treatment modalities with radiotherapy. © 2018 S. Karger AG, Basel

Role of the Tumor Microenvironment

The tumor microenvironment (TME) consists of multiple different structural and functional components, such as blood vessels, cancer-associated fibroblasts, bone marrow-derived inflammatory cells, lymphocytes, secreted signaling molecules, and the extracellular matrix (ECM). A variety of infiltrating myeloid cells, cancer-associated fibroblasts (CAFs), and angiogenic endothelial cells play critical functions in sustaining cell proliferation, evading growth suppressors, promoting tumor cell survival, activating invasion and dissemination, and reprogramming energy metabolism. In strong interaction with the heterogeneous tumor cell population, the TME thereby codefines the pathophysiology of the tumor [1].

Historically, drug discovery was primarily based on sensitivity studies on tumor cells and the identification of tumor cell-specific Achilles' heels, which could act as molecular-defined targets to increase a therapeutic window. This approach resulted in therapeutic successes, like clinically relevant inhibitors of the epidermal growth factor (EGF)-receptor tyrosine kinase (RTK) family, BCR-ABL-kinase, or ALK RTK in particular in tumor types, which are addicted to these pathways [2]. However, aggressive tumors grow in the interactive milieu of tumor cells with the multiple components of the TME. These interactions determine the potency of tumor cell-specific agents and at the same time reveal novel therapeutic approaches [3].

Tumor Hypoxia
Rapid and uncontrolled tumor proliferation results in a critical shortage of nutrients and oxygen, and subsequent adaptations of the tumor cells and the TME [4]. Tumor areas with limited oxygen supply remain a common feature throughout the lifetime of the tumor. Lack of oxygen in tumor areas primarily arises from oxygen consumption by vessel-proximal cells, oxygen diffusion limitations [5], and blood perfusion deficiencies, and is due to an insufficient or nonfunctional vasculature (diffusion-limited hypoxia and perfusion-limited hypoxia) [6]. Hypoxia is an adverse prognostic factor for patient outcome apart from tumor stage and nodal status [7]. Generally, hypoxic cells (<0.15 mm Hg) are more resistant to ionizing radiation (IR) as compared to normoxic cells by a factor of 2.5–3.0, i.e., up to 3 times higher doses of IR are required to produce equal cell killing [8].

The irradiation of cells leads to the formation of reactive oxygen species (ROS), which induce cytotoxic DNA damage. Furthermore, the oxygenation fixation theory implies that radiation-induced free radical sites in the DNA are chemically derivatized ("fixed") in the presence of oxygen so that they cannot be repaired and accumulate, leading to an enhanced rate of cell death. Thus, the intratumoral pO_2-heterogeneity translates to differences of several logs in cell killing between normoxic and hypoxic cells and is thereby a limiting factor for local tumor control by radiotherapy.

At the same time, several hypoxia-related transformation processes are induced at the cellular and tumor physiological level. Tumor hypoxia drives metabolic adaptation to a low oxygen content on the cellular level, alters DNA repair capacity via reduced expression of critical DNA repair and DNA damage response elements, thereby promoting genomic instability, and exerts a selection pressure towards a more aggressive phenotype. At low pO_2, genes involved in drug resistance are upregulated and confer resistance to various chemotherapeutic agents, such as the P-glycoprotein multidrug resistance protein. Furthermore, hypoxia drives the expression and secretion of several enzymes and chemo- and cytokines into the TME, resulting in an uncontrolled proangiogenic environment. As such, the gene-expression signature of the hypoxia response is a strong predictor of clinical outcomes, for example, in ovarian and breast cancers [9–11]. Besides extended efforts to generate noninvasive imaging-based approaches to determine the overall hypoxic status and to identify tumor subcompartments with a low oxygen content or altered metabolism, a strong interest also exists to identify predictive gene-hypoxia classifiers, like in head and neck squamous cell carcinoma. Such a genetically based classifier might lead towards more personalized hypoxia-oriented combined radiochemotherapy regimens [12–14].

Tumor Vasculature, Stromal Compartment, and ECM
The tumor vasculature is characterized by multiple structural and functional deficiencies, such as excessive vessel branching, erratic blood flow, and abnormal stromal proliferation [6]. Sprout-

ing angiogenesis, vasculogenesis through bone marrow-derived myeloid cells, and other modes of angiogenesis are relevant not only for tumor growth, but also for treatment sensitivity and recurrences [15]. Importantly, each endothelial cell supports almost 2,000 surrounding tumor cells. Therefore, the tumor vasculature and its genetic integrity represents an interesting therapeutic target. Apart from direct tumor cell killing, irradiation also damages and kills tumor endothelial cells, circulating endothelial cells, and bone marrow-derived endothelial progenitor cells. These antivascular effects contribute to the overall tumor response to radiotherapy.

The bidirectional interaction of tumor cells with the adjacent stromal cells is relevant for tumor growth, mechanical stability, and nutritional support. These stromal cells, which include endothelial cells, immune cells, fibroblasts, smooth muscle cells, adipocytes, and tissue stem cells, create and maintain the extracellular scaffold and compose the bulk of the TME. Stromal cells coevolve with tumor cells throughout tumorigenesis and their interactions promote tumor cell dissemination and create suitable metastatic niches [16]. The dynamic intercellular interactions are tightly controlled, for example by matrix metalloproteinases or reinforcement of collagen deposition. Indeed, the role of tumor stromal cells is emerging as a key factor determining tumor phenotype and treatment sensitivity [17]. For example, in pancreatic ductal adenocarcinoma, the admixture of tumor cells with profibrogenic pancreatic stromal cells (stellate cells) promotes tumor progression and dissemination in vivo and reduces the effectiveness of both chemo- and radiotherapy [18]. Stromal cells may also promote neoplastic progression through epithelial-to-mesenchymal transition in an integrin and cadherin-dependent manner [19].

The role of stromal cells and the TME in general for treatment sensitivity is increasingly becoming a key consideration for the development of novel anticancer therapeutics [20]. Progress in in vitro screening platforms as well as orthotopic and "orthometastatic" xenograft and syngeneic mouse models have enabled comprehensive characterization of the impact of the TME on therapeutic efficacy.

Besides the aggregation of the multiple different cellular populations, the ECM also dictates the tumor growth, phenotype, and therapeutic response. The ECM comprises both diffusible crosstalk and physical linkages among cells, influencing tissue architecture and functional coordination between neighboring cells. The direct cellular interactions with the ECM may further modulate radiation sensitivity. Moreover, irradiation itself can influence cellular adhesion to and interactions with the ECM, particularly via integrin receptors, which directly constitute the cell-ECM interface. IR can also induce β_1-integrin expression in several tumor types, with a resultant increase in cellular radioresistance [21]. Integrins are cell surface adhesion molecules that mediate intercellular and cellular to extracellular matrix interactions, and thereby control invasive processes. Mechanistically, the protein complex consisting of FAK and Erk1 mediates IR-induced prosurvival signals, which is effectively compromised by β_1-integrin and EGFR blocking [22]. Integrins also regulate downstream signal transduction cascades of the PI3K-AKT-NF-κB and MEK-ERK pathways. β_1-integrin overexpression enhances the phosphorylation of Akt-Ser473 and ERK1/2, and thereby triggers proliferative and survival pathways, bypassing the inhibitory effects of the upstream anti-HER2-directed antibody trastuzumab [23].

Tumor Microenvironment-Related Treatment Resistance

The bidirectional interplay between tumor and stroma cells is now considered as a prominent signature of cancer development [1]. Nonmalignant components of the tumor stromal microenvironment not only influence neoplastic growth and dissemination, but also codetermine the response to diverse treatment modalities, including micro-environment-mediated drug resistance [17, 24, 25], as clearly demonstrated on the preclinical level.

The primary cytotoxic target of IR-generated ROS is DNA, profoundly affecting the cellular genetic integrity, both in tumor cells, tumor-associated stromal cells, and in the coirradiated normal tissue. In addition, ROS also induce multiple systemic and intracellular stress responses independent of the DNA damage, but via a variety of proteins with built-in sensors for oxidation. Thereby, radiotherapy affects the qualitative and quantitative composition of the TME and the intercellular communication, via the secretion of regulatory molecules that stimulate or inhibit cellular proliferation and differentiation.

Autocrine and paracrine signaling are induced by various secreted factors, which maintain the activation of multiple intracellular signal transduction cascades and mediate treatment resistance. These factors support the formation of a "treatment-resistant or metastatic niche" and act as a reservoir for subsequent relapses [26]. A prominent example represents IR- and hypoxia-enhanced secretion of lysyl oxidase (LOX). LOX is a cell-secreted amine oxidase that crosslinks collagen and elastin in the extracellular space, and plays an important role in hypoxia-dependent cancer cell dissemination and metastasis. Elevated expression of tumor-derived LOX is associated with metastasis and poor survival in lung, mammary, and head and neck cancer patients [27–30]. Work by others and in part from our own research demonstrated that the activity of matrix metalloproteases and LOX, key regulators of the ECM, are activated or secreted in response to hypoxia and IR, and thereby contributes to an invasive phenotype.

Tumor Vasculature-Related Treatment Resistance

Apart from direct tumor cell killing, radiotherapy acts on the level of the tumor vasculature, damaging and killing tumor endothelial cells, circulating endothelial cells and bone marrow-derived endothelial progenitor cells, leading to the dose-dependent destruction of blood vessels and subsequent endothelial cell dysfunction [6]. Irradiation induces drastic vessel permeability, detachment of endothelial cells from the basement membrane, and programmed cell death. Interestingly, upregulation of acid sphingomyelinases, ASMase, in response to a high single-fraction dose (8–16 Gy) was demonstrated to result in endothelial cell death, inflammation, and fibrosis. These original data on the role of the acidic sphingomyelinase in the tumor endothelial cells suggest that the radiation sensitivity of the tumor vasculature codetermines the overall outcome, in particular in response to single high-dose irradiation [31]. Even though the involvement of the bone marrow as part of these studies has not been sufficiently clarified so far, they nevertheless prompted the field of combining radiotherapy with inhibitors of angiogenesis, also radiosensitizing the tumor vasculature (see below).

In comparison to the vasculature in healthy tissue, tumor endothelial cells rapidly proliferate, which contribute to their enhanced radiation sensitivity. Vascular damages in response to high-dose radiotherapy leads to chronic hypoxia and increased secretion of cytokines, chemokines, and angiogenic factors that can induce immune cell recruitment. Subsequent vascular normalization is driven in a hypoxia-inducible factor 1α (HIF-1α)-dependent manner with a subsequently enhanced production of VEGFA, PDGFA, and others, and HIF-1α-independent mechanisms, including the recruitment of bone marrow-derived cells [5, 15, 32, 33].

Endothelial cells may also directly secrete biologically active factors thereby shaping the tumor response to cytotoxic treatment modalities. For example, in the Burkitt lymphoma mouse model, the prosurvival factors IL-6 and TIMP-1 are secreted from thymic endothelial cells in response to doxorubicin and thereby create a "chemoresistant niche" in the TME, increasing lymphoma cell survival and eventual relapse [26]. Likewise, endothelial cells can also promote a cancer stem cell phenotype in colorectal tumors via the secretion of Jagged-1 and eventually Notch activation [34].

Tumor cell-linked chemotherapy-resistance might also lead to an ineffective antiangiogenic response, for example in the case of strongly enhanced secretion of proangiogenic factors, which is not anymore abrogated by the chemotherapeutic agent. Therefore, combining a cytotoxic agent with vasculature-targeting agents can resensitize the treatment-resistant tumor. Our own studies demonstrated that a combined treatment modality of microtubule-interfering agents (MIA) with inhibitors of angiogenesis such as VEGFA-directed antibodies or mTOR inhibitors can overcome tumor cell-linked MIA resistance in different tumor models, derived from genetically defined MIA-resistant lung and colon adenocarcinoma tumor cells [35]. As such, therapeutic interventions lead to the unanticipated creation of distinct niches that are seeds for recurrences and limit their efficacies.

Tumor Cell-Driven Treatment Resistance
Tumor cell-mediated resistance involves the secretion of tumor cell-derived survival factors in response to irradiation, which act in an auto- and paracrine way. For example, IR induces the secretion of IL-6 [36], transforming growth factor-beta 1 (TGF-β1) [37], IL-8 [38], COX2 (cyclooxygenase 2) [39], and tumor necrosis factor alpha (TNF-α) [39]. These factors result in a transient or prolonged activation of respective survival thresholds and support the outgrowth of radioresistant tumor subclones [40].

Furthermore, prominent survival factors that are induced by IR are multiple ligands of the EGF family [41], proinflammatory cytokines [42–44], fibroblast growth factor TGF-β [45], VEGFA [46], stromal cell-derived factor-1 (SDF-1) [47], and many others. For example, radiotherapy also upregulates expression of the key angiogenic mediator PDGF, leading to phosphorylation of the PDGF receptor. This IR-mediated phosphorylation can be strongly inhibited by PDGF-tyrosine kinase inhibitors [48]. Similarly, thoracic irradiation increases serum levels of TGF-β1, promoting circulating tumor cells and lung dissemination, which can be antagonized by a specific neutralizing pan-TGF-β antibody [49].

VEGFA-secretion is upregulated in response to radiotherapy across multiple cell lines in vitro and in vivo [46]. IR also induces expression of HIF-1 and SDF-1 at the tumor invasion front, which is associated with enhanced tumor infiltration by tumor-associated macrophages, TAMs, leading to tumor revascularization [47]. Low-dose radiotherapy can induce G-CSF protein and GM-CSF mRNA expression, resulting in the recruitment of progenitor cells from peripheral blood [50]. Our own findings demonstrate that radiotherapy can induce the secretion of multiple ADAM17 substrates such as ALCAM and amphiregulin in the TME. Genetic or pharmacologic targeting of ADAM17 activity can subsequently sensitize NSCLC tumors to radiotherapy (see below) [51].

Fibrotic Compartment-Linked Treatment Resistance
Besides fibrosis-linked normal tissue complications, fibroblast-mediated resistance also codetermines the treatment outcome. Anticancer agents including IR lead to the secretion of multiple factors from fibroblasts, which support neoplastic progression in vivo. Soluble mediators released by irradiated fibroblasts stimulate primary tumor growth and the invasive potential of cancer cells through upregulation of c-Met expression and MAP kinase activity [52, 53]. CAFs secrete ECM components (such as tenascin C and collagen I), matrix-modifying enzymes (MMP2, 9, and 13), and cytokines (HGF, CXCL12, and PDGF), and thereby activate tumor cell survival signaling in a paracrine way. CAFs are relatively

radiation resistant and have a mesenchymal morphology. As such, patient-derived human lung CAFs survive ablative doses of radiation but interestingly loose part of their invasive phenotype postirradiation. This might be linked to the stabilization of adhesive integrins such as β_1-integrin [54]. Likewise, pancreatic fibroblasts render pancreatic tumor cells more radiation resistant to single high doses and fractionated doses of IR. Abrogating β_1-integrin signaling abolishes the pancreatic fibroblast-mediated radioprotective effect in a PI3K (phosphoinositide 3-kinase) independent but FAK-dependent manner [55].

Immune-Driven Radiation Resistance
The immune compartment also represents an important part of the TME, which affects the clinical response and resistance. Of note, a strong interest currently exists to gain detailed insights on the interface of radiotherapy and immunology. These aspects, including the development of novel combined treatment modalities with immune checkpoints inhibitors, are discussed in a separate chapter of this book.

Targeting Microenvironment-Mediated Radioresistance

There is compelling evidence that the TME can mediate resistance to radiotherapy and is a crucial determinant of therapeutic efficacy (see above) [5]. The efficacy of radiotherapy can be improved by cooperative targeting combining irradiation with agents targeting different compartments of the TME or with secretome-targeting agents derived from the irradiated tumor or stromal cell.

Targeting the Tumor Cell Compartment
The tumor cell compartment is the primary target of radiotherapy and irreparable or misrepaired DNA damage is the major cytotoxic effect of IR. In addition, IR-generated ROS trigger an intracellular stress response resulting in the modulation of multiple intracellular pathways and secretion of various autocrine and paracrine factors. These secreted factors eventually codetermine the tumor response to irradiation and dictate the treatment outcome. For example, IR-induced phosphorylation of the PDGF-receptor is strongly inhibited by PDGF-RTK inhibitors leading to substantial tumor growth control [48]. Thoracic irradiation increases serum levels of TGF-β_1, circulating tumor cells, and lung metastases, which can be antagonized by specific neutralizing pan-TGF-β antibodies [49]. Similarly, VEGF expression and secretion is induced in response to irradiation and its inhibition by VEGF-directed neutralizing antibodies, small-molecular VEGF-RTK-inhibitors, or dominant-negative soluble receptors inhibit primary tumor growth and invasion across a broad range of tumor models [46, 56, 57].

Instead of targeting individual factors, a more promising approach might represent the targeting of common upstream enzymes that are processing multiple survival factors. Our own work demonstrated such an approach both in vitro and in vivo: IR activates the matrix metalloproteinase ADAM17 via a dose-dependent increase of furin-mediated cleavage of the proform of ADAM17 to active ADAM17. IR-induced ADAM17 activity results in enhanced secretion of multiple ADAM17 ligands into the microenvironment. Interestingly, targeting of ADAM17 activity enhances IR-induced cytotoxicity at the level of clonogenic survival, which suggests that modulation of ADAM17 activity and subsequent downstream factors not only act on the paracrine, but also in a autocrine way at the tumor cell level [51]. Radiotherapy also induces the secretion of multiple ADAM17-cleaved EGFR ligands – as demonstrated on the preclinical and clinical level – such as TGF-α, amphiregulin, EGF, and others [58, 59]. As such, ADAM17 is a promising target as inhibition of its proteolytic activity not only affects a single RTK, for example the EGFR, and its downstream signal transduction cascades, but

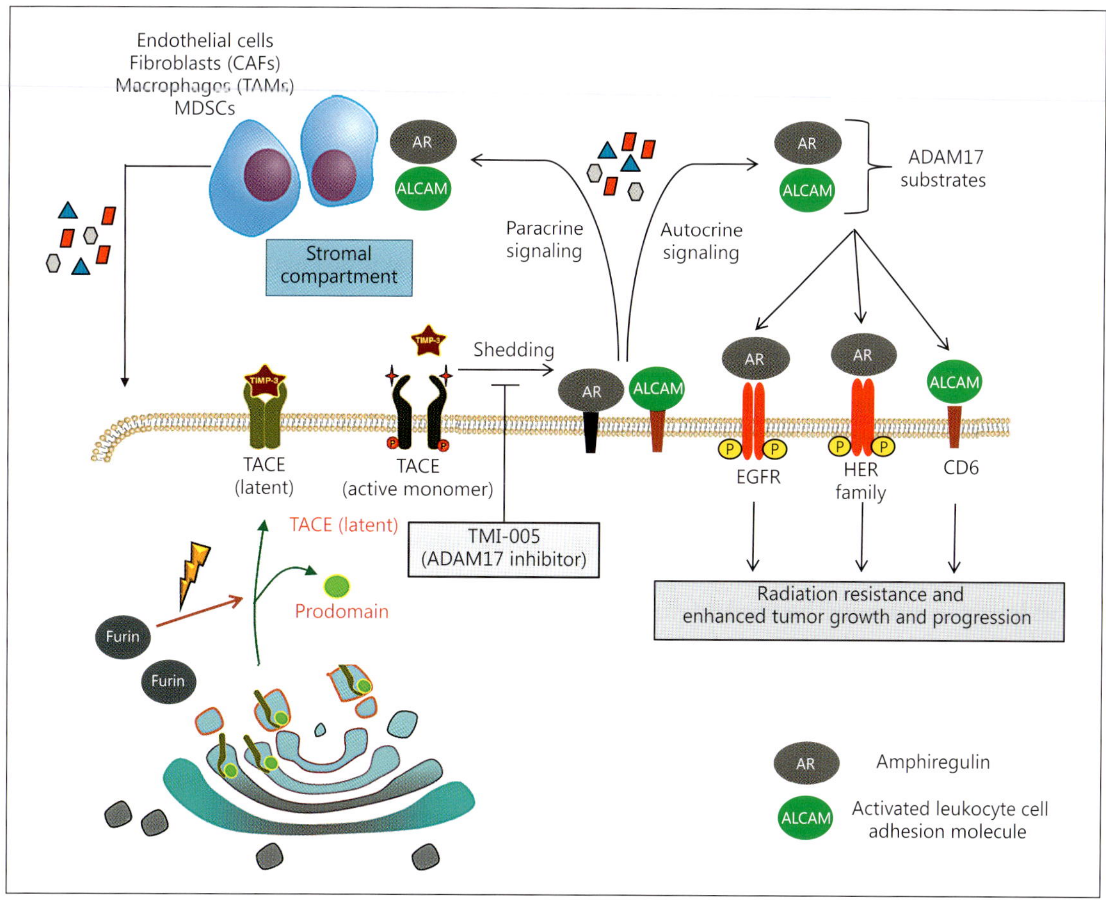

Fig. 1. Radiosensitization of non-small-cell lung cancer by targeting IR-induced activation of ADAM17. Radiotherapy leads to the secretion of multiple ADAM17 substrates such as ALCAM, amphiregulin, and TGF-α into the tumor microenvironment. Genetic or pharmacologic targeting of ADAM17 suppresses (IR-induced) shedding of secreted factors and thereby affects auto- and paracrine effects of ADAM17-shed factors [51, 60].

also deregulates multiple auto- and paracrine-controlled processes, resulting in broad antitumor potency both in EGFR ligand-dependent and EGFR ligand-independent tumors [60] (Fig. 1).

Targeting Tumor Hypoxia: Hypoxic Radiosensitizers and Hypoxia-Activated Prodrugs
Several strategies have been developed during recent decades to overcome the hurdle of tumor hypoxia for successful radiotherapy. These strategies can be grouped into fundamentally different approaches. While hypoxic radiosensitizers and bioreductive cytotoxics are preferentially effective in hypoxic parts of the tumor, other classes of agents, including the various inhibitors of angiogenesis, aim to increase oxygen availability in the tumor and subsequently to reduce tumor hypoxia and radiation resistance.

The prototype of hypoxic radiosensitizers are the electron-affinic nitroimidazoles, such as misonidazole, etanidazole, pimonidazole, and the clinically approved nimorazole, which is given as standard of care in patients for head and

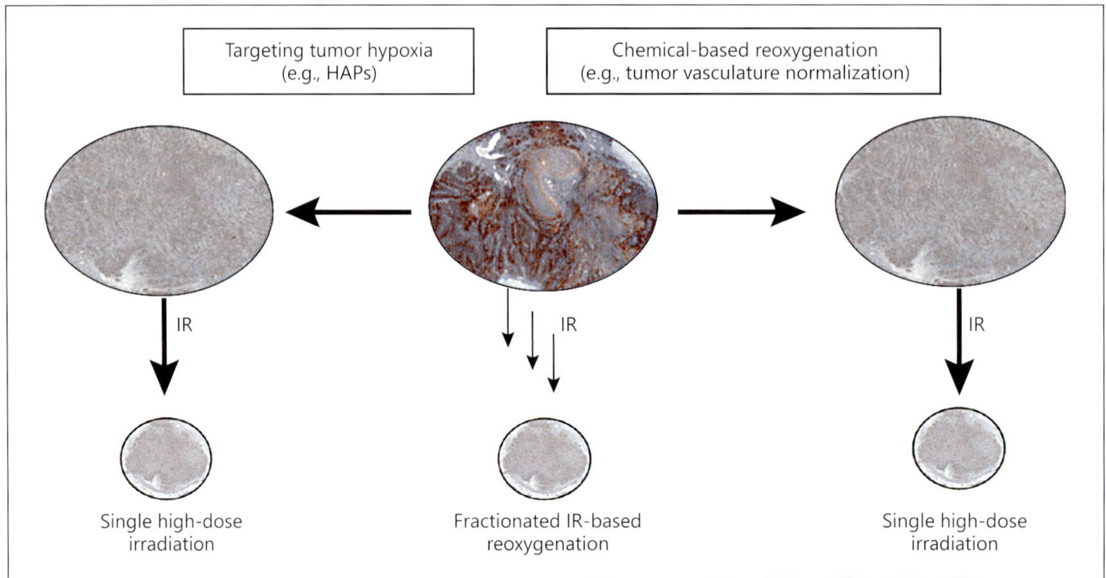

Fig. 2. Multiple approaches to overcome tumor hypoxia as a major challenge for radiotherapy reoxygenation of the hypoxic tumor compartment can be achieved by fractionated low-dose irradiation alone. Single high-dose IR can be combined with pharmaceutical agents either specifically targeting tumor hypoxia (e.g., with hypoxia-activated prodrugs) or inducing biology-based tumor reoxygenation (see text for details).

stabilize leaky vessels, and to remodel the dysfunctional tumor vasculature to a normal phenotype with increased tumor blood flow and oxygen delivery. This process could contribute to the increased treatment response originally observed and now aimed for by the combined treatment modality of IR with inhibitors of angiogenesis. However, a major obstacle is that normalization of the tumor vasculature is a transient process only occurring within a short time window and highly dependent on the correct dosing of the respective inhibitor and on the individual tumor environment [6, 35, 84, 85].

Nevertheless, an enhanced radiation response could be demonstrated in several preclinical studies when tumors were irradiated during a transient increase of tumor oxygenation [86, 87]. These studies were performed on tumor xenografts and orthotopic tumor models treated with different classes of antiangiogenic agents, such as the VEGF-directed antibody Avastin, the VEGF receptor-directed antibody DC-101, the antiangiogenic peptide Anginex, or multiple VEGF-RTK inhibitors [81, 88–91]. Furthermore, not only endothelial-directed compounds, but also tumor cell signaling- directed agents may contribute to a window of tumor vasculature normalization, for example by the reduction of VEGF secretion, leading to reduced radiation resistance [90, 92, 93].

Inhibitors of angiogenesis were also shown to increase tumor hypoxia in tumor xenografts and in spontaneous murine tumor models, which might result in enhanced radiation resistance [94, 95]. However, the inhibitor of angiogenesis-increased tumor hypoxia is most probably nullified when combined with irradiation, presumably due to the decreased demand for oxygen by the drastically reduced number of tumor cells surviving the first few fractions of irradiation [95].

Pharmacological-induced normalization of the tumor vasculature with concomitant reoxygenation is an interesting concept. However, a fractionated treatment regimen of IR with concomitant IR-induced reoxygenation might even supersede this effect. We currently cannot predict which tumor entities and phenotypes will respond to antiangiogenic compounds accordingly, not even on the preclinical experimental level. Even more challenges exist in the clinic before a defined window of tumor vasculature normalization could be identified on the individual patient situation, for example using hypoxia PET imaging, to be exploited for stereotactic body radiation therapy.

Conflicting data on the outcome of different treatment regimens exist when using inhibitors of angiogenesis in combination with IR. Overall, it is not a neoadjuvant but rather a concomitant and even more so an adjuvant treatment regimen that results in an enhanced tumor response to irradiation in combination with several investigated antiangiogenic compounds [80, 81, 96–99]. As such, preclinical scheduling experiments suggest additional mechanisms to contribute to radiosensitization by antiangiogenic agents, besides normalization of the tumor vasculature. IR affects the tumor vasculature in multiple ways, including the switch to other forms of angiogenesis (see below) [100, 101]. However, irradiation also induces endothelial cell apoptosis, and the apoptotic response on the level of the tumor vasculature correlates with the tumor response to single high doses of IR ($>$15 Gy) [31]. Inhibitors of angiogenesis also induce endothelial cell apoptosis and thus, independent of their potential to induce a window of tumor vasculature normalization and even applied in an adjuvant regimen, might enhance the fragility of the tumor vasculature also to low-dose fractions of irradiation, and thereby increase the efficacy of radiotherapy [102–104].

Tumor hypoxia can be regarded as a shifted balance between demand and supply of oxygen relative to the normal tissue. Several earlier strategies were developed to increase the oxygen transport capacity of the blood and perfusion of the tumor with more oxygen, which include hy-perbaric oxygen therapy, blood transfusion in anemic patients, or accelerated radiotherapy with carbogen and nicotinamide, ARCON [105–107]. An increase of the hemoglobin concentration could also be achieved by erythropoietin injections, but clinical studies revealed increased radiation resistance upon erythropoietin, which can be linked to radiation-protective erythropoietin-induced signaling in tumor cells [108, 109].

Rapidly proliferating tumors and aberrant vasculature lead to both acute and chronic hypoxia. Treating these tumors with radiotherapy results in an altered microenvironment and cycling hypoxia. Inhibiting VEGFA with the VEGF-specific antibody bevacizumab can sensitize tumors to radiotherapy through a reduction of hypoxia [6]. The clinical effects of bevacizumab are short lived, and therefore targeting downstream molecules such as PI3K and mTOR in combination with radiotherapy can result in effective long-term vasculature normalization and a durable clinical response. Similarly, the dual inhibitor of PI3K and mTOR, NVP-BEZ235, can result in additive tumor growth delay when combined with irradiation, as it improves tumor oxygenation and vasculature over a prolonged period [92]. Endostar, a novel recombinant human endostatin radiosensitizes cancer cells by inhibiting TGF-β_1 [110], VEGF, and KDR downstream signaling [111], and is currently being investigated in combination with radiotherapy in phase II clinical trials. Recurrence postradiotherapy might be mediated by the recruitment of bone marrow-derived progenitor cells in a VEGFA- and angiopoietin2-dependent manner. Inhibition of ANG2 can overcome resistance to anti-VEGF therapies and prevent recurrences postradiotherapy [112].

Vasculogenesis represents an additional form of tumor vasculature generation. Glioblastoma tumor recurrences could be linked to vasculogenesis instead of sprouting angiogenesis from the irradiated tumor bed. Posttreatment vasculogenesis is promoted via local secretion of the SDF-1 signaling axis recruiting bone marrow-derived cells into the irradiated tumor site. Interestingly, blocking the SDF-1-CXCR4-receptor interaction with plerixafor strongly reduced tumor recurrences after radiotherapy in orthotopic tumor models and is already being tested in the clinical setting [101, 113]. Likewise, matrix metalloproteinase-9 produced by bone marrow-derived CD11b+ myelomonocytic cells allows tumors to grow in irradiated normal tissues of the mice, and therefore targeting of MMP-9 sensitizes tumors to radiotherapy [114].

Targeting Tumor Metabolism

Novel approaches focus on the reduction of the oxygen demand, based on gained insights on the tumor metabolism. Besides hypoxic tumor cells and tumor cells adapted to aerobic glycolysis by the Warburg effect, a major proportion of cells in the tumor still use oxidative phosphorylation with a high rate of oxygen consumption as a source of energy. Therefore, compounds shifting cells to aerobic glycolysis or directly targeting mitochondrial respiration and metabolism, for example with arsenic trioxide, sensitize for IR-induced cytotoxic DNA damage by creating (a window of) enhanced tumor oxygenation due to reduced oxygen consumption [115–117]. Interestingly, tumor cells fuel oxidative phosphorylation not only from glucose in the blood, but primarily from lactate after cellular uptake by the lactate transporter MCT1 and oxidation of lactate to pyruvate by lactate dehydrogenase. This leaves sufficient glucose for ATP generation of hypoxic tumor cells by glycolysis and for tumor cells adapted to aerobic glycolysis [118]. Pharmacologic inhibition of the respective lactate transporter MCT1 results in a switch from lactate-fueled respiration to glucose-fueled aerobic glycolysis in these tumor cells. Therefore, glucose availability becomes limited for hypoxic cells below a critical threshold for survival. At the same time, oxygen in the tumor is spared by an overall reduced oxidative phosphorylation in the tumor, and subsequent tumor reoxygenation sensitizes

for a single high-dose treatment with IR. These novel insights on the hallmark of tumor metabolism might indeed create innovative approaches for radiosensitization with a high translational potential.

Targeting the Fibrotic Compartment

The fibroblast compartment comprises CAFs, which influence long-term fibrotic processes and tumor recurrences. Radiotherapy leads to the upregulation of the proinflammatory NF-κB pathway in CAFs that further enhances the expression and secretion of the cytokines TGF-β1, IL-1β, IL-6, IL-8, and GM-CSF into the TME. A radiation resistance-promoting phenotype is also induced by CAF-secreted HGF (hepatocyte growth factor) and the glycoprotein TNC (Tenascin-C), which is expressed in the ECM. Irradiation of tumor cells leads to the overexpression of the HGF-RTK MET and thereby might adapt a more invasive phenotype via a HGF-MET-dependent mechanism. Genetic or pharmacological targeting of MET signaling by siRNA or specific MET kinase inhibitors such as PHA665752 or JNJ-38877605 inhibit radiation-induced proliferation and invasiveness, and promote radiation-induced cytotoxicity as investigated in mammary carcinoma and glioblastoma cells [119]. Likewise, the invasiveness of pancreatic cancer cells is augmented by co-culturing with irradiated fibroblasts. This fibroblast-induced invasiveness is counteracted by NK4, a specific antagonist of HGF [52]. ^{131}I-labeled TNC-specific antibodies, such as 81C6 and F16SIP, effectively target CAF-derived tenascin. In a phase II trial, ^{131}I-labeled 81C6 demonstrated better median survival as compared to the classic radio-chemotherapeutic regimen irrespective of the prognostic markers and revealed survival benefits, although with acute toxicities [120, 121]. Even though targeting the fibroblast compartment remains in its infancy, its genetic stability as compared to the tumor cell compartment makes it an attractive target in combination with radiotherapy.

The genetic instability of the tumor cell compartment with concomitant differential treatment resistances represents a major challenge for successful radiotherapy alone and as part of combined treatment modalities. Furthermore, tumor heterogeneity also derives from the complex interactions of tumor cells with the stromal compartment that determine a distinct TME on the individual tumor level. However, and despite intense and decade-long research, for example in the field of tumor hypoxia, we are only now starting to understand how the different cellular entities and compartments in a tumor communicate with each other and thereby govern tumor growth and treatment resistance. At the same time, these dynamic and even treatment-induced interactions within the tumor represent promising targets for novel combined treatment modalities with radiotherapy.

References

1 Junttila MR, de Sauvage FJ: Influence of tumour micro-environment heterogeneity on therapeutic response. Nature 2013;501:346–354.

2 Tandon R, et al: Dual epidermal growth factor receptor (EGFR)/insulin-like growth factor-1 receptor (IGF-1R) inhibitor: a novel approach for overcoming resistance in anticancer treatment. Eur J Pharmacol 2011;667:56–65.

3 Barker HE, Paget JT, Khan AA, Harrington KJ: The tumour microenvironment after radiotherapy: mechanisms of resistance and recurrence. Nat Rev Cancer 2015;15:409–425.

4 Fluegen G, et al: Phenotypic heterogeneity of disseminated tumour cells is preset by primary tumour hypoxic microenvironments. Nat Cell Biol 2017;19:120–132.

5 Begg AC, Stewart FA, Vens C: Strategies to improve radiotherapy with targeted drugs. Nat Rev Cancer 2011;11:239–253.

6 Jain RK: Normalization of tumor vasculature: an emerging concept in antiangiogenic therapy. Science (New York) 2005;307:58–62.

7 Vaupel P, Mayer A: Hypoxia in cancer: significance and impact on clinical outcome. Cancer Metastasis Rev 2007;26:225–239.

8 Wouters BG, Brown JM: Cells at intermediate oxygen levels can be more important than the "hypoxic fraction" in determining tumor response to fractionated radiotherapy. Radiat Res 1997;147:541–550.

9 Chi JT, et al: Gene expression programs in response to hypoxia: cell type specificity and prognostic significance in human cancers. PLoS Med 2006;3:e47.

10 Graeber TG, et al: Hypoxia-mediated selection of cells with diminished apoptotic potential in solid tumours. Nature 1996;379:88–91.

11 Chan N, et al: Chronic hypoxia decreases synthesis of homologous recombination proteins to offset chemoresistance and radioresistance. Cancer Res 2008;68:605–614.

12 Toustrup K, et al: Validation of a 15-gene hypoxia classifier in head and neck cancer for prospective use in clinical trials. Acta Oncol 2016;55:1091–1098.

13 Toustrup K, Sorensen BS, Alsner J, Overgaard J: Hypoxia gene expression signatures as prognostic and predictive markers in head and neck radiotherapy. Semin Radiat Oncol 2012;22:119–127.

14 Harris BH, Barberis A, West CM, Buffa FM: Gene expression signatures as biomarkers of tumour hypoxia. Clin Oncol 2015;27:547–560.

15 Ahn GO, Brown JM: Influence of bone marrow-derived hematopoietic cells on the tumor response to radiotherapy: experimental models and clinical perspectives. Cell Cycle (Georgetown) 2009;8:970–976.

16 Mlecnik B, et al: The tumor microenvironment and Immunoscore are critical determinants of dissemination to distant metastasis. Sci Transl Med 2016;8:327ra326.

17 McMillin DW, et al: Tumor cell-specific bioluminescence platform to identify stroma-induced changes to anticancer drug activity. Nat Med 2010;16:483–489.

18 Hwang RF, et al: Cancer-associated stromal fibroblasts promote pancreatic tumor progression. Cancer Res 2008;68:918–926.

19 Kikuta K, et al: Pancreatic stellate cells promote epithelial-mesenchymal transition in pancreatic cancer cells. Biochem Biophys Res Commun 2010;403:380–384.

20 Dart A: Tumour microenvironment: genotype puts tension on a tumour. Nat Rev Cancer 2016;16:341.

21 Eke I, et al: Simultaneous beta1 integrin-EGFR targeting and radiosensitization of human head and neck cancer. J Natl Cancer Inst 2015;107:dju419.

22 Eke I, et al: β_1 integrin/FAK/cortactin signaling is essential for human head and neck cancer resistance to radiotherapy. J Clin Invest 2012;122:1529–1540.

23 Lesniak D, et al: β_1-integrin circumvents the antiproliferative effects of trastuzumab in human epidermal growth factor receptor-2-positive breast cancer. Cancer Res 2009;69:8620–8628.

24 Kannaiyan R, et al: Celastrol inhibits proliferation and induces chemosensitization through down-regulation of NF-κB and STAT3 regulated gene products in multiple myeloma cells. Br J Pharmacol 2011;164:1506–1521.

25 Obenauf AC, et al: Therapy-induced tumour secretomes promote resistance and tumour progression. Nature 2015;520:368–372.

26 Gilbert LA, Hemann MT: DNA damage-mediated induction of a chemoresistant niche. Cell 2010;143:355–366.

27 Barker HE, Cox TR, Erler JT: The rationale for targeting the LOX family in cancer. Nat Rev Cancer 2012;12:540–552.

28 Cox TR, et al: The hypoxic cancer secretome induces pre-metastatic bone lesions through lysyl oxidase. Nature 2015;522:106–110.

29 Erler JT, et al: Lysyl oxidase is essential for hypoxia-induced metastasis. Nature 2006;440:1222–1226.

30 Shen CJ, et al: Ionizing radiation induces tumor cell lysyl oxidase secretion. BMC Cancer 2014;14:532.

31 Garcia-Barros M, et al: Tumor response to radiotherapy regulated by endothelial cell apoptosis. Science (New York) 2003; 300:1155–1159.

32 Kozin, S. V, et al: Recruitment of myeloid but not endothelial precursor cells facilitates tumor regrowth after local irradiation. Cancer Res 2010;70:5679–5685.

33 Lerman OZ, et al: Low-dose radiation augments vasculogenesis signaling through HIF-1-dependent and -independent SDF-1 induction. Blood 2010; 116:3669–3676.

34 Lu J, et al: Endothelial cells promote the colorectal cancer stem cell phenotype through a soluble form of Jagged-1. Cancer Cell 2013;23:171–185.

35 Broggini-Tenzer A, et al: Combined treatment strategies for microtubule stabilizing agent-resistant tumors. J Natl Cancer Inst 2015;107:dju504.

36 Chou CH, et al: Radiation-induced hepatitis B virus reactivation in liver mediated by the bystander effect from irradiated endothelial cells. Clin Cancer Res 2007;13:851–857.

37 Iyer R, Lehnert BE, Svensson R: Factors underlying the cell growth-related bystander responses to alpha particles. Cancer Res 2000;60:1290–1298.

38 Narayanan PK, LaRue KE, Goodwin EH, Lehnert BE: Alpha particles induce the production of interleukin-8 by human cells. Radiat Res 1999;152:57–63.

39 Zhou H, et al: Mechanism of radiation-induced bystander effect: role of the cyclooxygenase-2 signaling pathway. Proc Natl Acad Sci USA 2005;102: 14641–14646.

40 Bentzen SM, Harari PM, Bernier J: Exploitable mechanisms for combining drugs with radiation: concepts, achievements and future directions. Nat Clin Pract Oncol 2007;4:172–180.

41 Dent P, Yacoub A, Fisher PB, Hagan MP, Grant S: MAPK pathways in radiation responses. Oncogene 2003;22: 5885–5896.

42 McBride WH, et al: A sense of danger from radiation. Radiat Res 2004;162: 1–19.

43 Neta R: Modulation of radiation damage by cytokines. Stem Cells (Dayton) 1997; 15(suppl 2):87–94.

44 Han SK, Song JY, Yun YS, Yi SY: Effect of gamma radiation on cytokine expression and cytokine-receptor mediated STAT activation. Int J Radiat Biol 2006; 82:686–697.

45 Barcellos-Hoff MH, Derynck R, Tsang ML, Weatherbee JA: Transforming growth factor-beta activation in irradiated murine mammary gland. J Clin Invest 1994;93:892–899.

46 Gorski DH, et al: Blockage of the vascular endothelial growth factor stress response increases the antitumor effects of ionizing radiation. Cancer Res 1999;59: 3374–3378.

47 Wang SC, Yu CF, Hong JH, Tsai CS, Chiang CS: Radiation therapy-induced tumor invasiveness is associated with SDF-1-regulated macrophage mobilization and vasculogenesis. PloS One 2013; 8:e69182.

48 Abdollahi A, et al: Inhibition of platelet-derived growth factor signaling attenuates pulmonary fibrosis. J Exp Med 2005;201:925–935.

49 Biswas S, et al: Inhibition of TGF-β with neutralizing antibodies prevents radiation-induced acceleration of metastatic cancer progression. J Clin Invest 2007; 117:1305–1313.

50 Li W, Wang G, Cui J, Xue L, Cai L: Low-dose radiation (LDR) induces hematopoietic hormesis: LDR-induced mobilization of hematopoietic progenitor cells into peripheral blood circulation. Exp Hematol 2004;32:1088–1096.

51 Sharma A, et al: Secretome signature identifies ADAM17 as novel target for radiosensitization of non-small cell lung cancer. Clin Cancer Res 2016;22:4428–4439.

52 Ohuchida K, et al: Radiation to stromal fibroblasts increases invasiveness of pancreatic cancer cells through tumor-stromal interactions. Cancer Res 2004; 64:3215–3222.

53 Barcellos-Hoff MH, Ravani SA: Irradiated mammary gland stroma promotes the expression of tumorigenic potential by unirradiated epithelial cells. Cancer Res 2000;60:1254–1260.

54 Hellevik T, et al: Cancer-associated fibroblasts from human NSCLC survive ablative doses of radiation but their invasive capacity is reduced. Radiat Oncol (London) 2012;7:59.

55 Mantoni TS, Lunardi S, Al-Assar O, Masamune A, Brunner TB: Pancreatic stellate cells radioprotect pancreatic cancer cells through beta1-integrin signaling. Cancer Res 2011;71:3453–3458.

56 Park JS, et al: Ionizing radiation modulates vascular endothelial growth factor (VEGF) expression through multiple mitogen activated protein kinase dependent pathways. Oncogene 2001;20: 3266–3280.

57 Williams KJ, et al: Combining radiotherapy with AZD2171, a potent inhibitor of vascular endothelial growth factor signaling: pathophysiologic effects and therapeutic benefit. Mol Cancer Ther 2007;6:599–606.

58 Hagan, M, Yacoub, A, Dent, P: Ionizing radiation causes a dose-dependent release of transforming growth factor alpha in vitro from irradiated xenografts and during palliative treatment of hormone-refractory prostate carcinoma. Clin Cancer Res 2004;10:5724–5731.

59 Toulany M, Baumann M, Rodemann HP: Stimulated PI3K-AKT signaling mediated through ligand or radiation-induced EGFR depends indirectly, but not directly, on constitutive K-Ras activity. Mol Cancer Res 2007;5:863–872.

60 Ieguchi K, Maru Y: Savior or not: ADAM17 inhibitors overcome radiotherapy-resistance in non-small cell lung cancer. J Thorac Dis 2016;8:E813–E815.

61 Overgaard J: Hypoxic modification of radiotherapy in squamous cell carcinoma of the head and neck–a systematic review and meta-analysis. Radiother Oncol 2011;100:22–32.

62 Adams GE, Cooke MS: Electron-affinic sensitization. I. A structural basis for chemical radiosensitizers in bacteria. Int J Radiat Biol Relat Stud Phys Chem Med 1969;15:457–471.

63 Horsman MR, Mortensen LS, Petersen JB, Busk M, Overgaard J: Imaging hypoxia to improve radiotherapy outcome. Nat Rev Clin Oncol 2012;9:674–687.

64 Brown JM: Keynote address: hypoxic cell radiosensitizers: where next? Int J Radiat Oncol Biol Phys 1989;16:987–993.

65 Denekamp J, Stewart FA: Sensitization of mouse tumours using fractionated X-irradiation. Br J Cancer 1978;3:259–263.

66 Overgaard J: Clinical evaluation of nitro-imidazoles as modifiers of hypoxia in solid tumors. Oncol Res 1994;6:509–518.

67 Mohindra JK, Rauth AM: Increased cell killing by metronidazole and nitrofurazone of hypoxic compared to aerobic mammalian cells. Cancer Res 1976;36:930–936.

68 Ahn GO, Brown M: Targeting tumors with hypoxia-activated cytotoxins. Front Biosci 2007;12:3483–3501.

69 Wilson WR, Hay MP: Targeting hypoxia in cancer therapy. Nat Rev Cancer 2011;11:393–410.

70 Liu Q, et al: TH-302, a hypoxia-activated prodrug with broad in vivo preclinical combination therapy efficacy: optimization of dosing regimens and schedules. Cancer Chemother Pharmacol 2012;69:1487–1498.

71 McKeage MJ, et al: PR-104 a bioreductive pre-prodrug combined with gemcitabine or docetaxel in a phase Ib study of patients with advanced solid tumours. BMC Cancer 2012;12:496.

72 Sun JD, et al: Selective tumor hypoxia targeting by hypoxia-activated prodrug TH-302 inhibits tumor growth in preclinical models of cancer. Clin Cancer Res 2012;18:758–770.

73 Meng F, et al: Molecular and cellular pharmacology of the hypoxia-activated prodrug TH-302. Mol Cancer Ther 2012;11:740–751.

74 Peeters SG, et al: TH-302 in combination with radiotherapy enhances the therapeutic outcome and is associated with pretreatment [^{18}F]HX4 hypoxia PET imaging. Clin Cancer Res 2015;21:2984–2992.

75 Yoon C, et al: Hypoxia-activated chemotherapeutic TH-302 enhances the effects of VEGF-A inhibition and radiation on sarcomas. Br J Cancer 2015;113:46–56.

76 Larue RT, et al: A phase 1 "window-of-opportunity" trial testing evofosfamide (TH-302), a tumour-selective hypoxia-activated cytotoxic prodrug, with preoperative chemoradiotherapy in oesophageal adenocarcinoma patients. BMC Cancer 2016;16:644.

77 Parveen I, Naughton DP, Whish WJ, Threadgill MD: 2-nitroimidazol-5-yl-methyl as a potential bioreductively activated prodrug system: reductively triggered release of the PARP inhibitor 5-bromoisoquinolinone. Bioorg Med Chem Lett 1999;9:2031–2036.

78 Thomson, P, et al: Synthesis and biological properties of bioreductively targeted nitrothienyl prodrugs of combretastatin A-4. Mol Cancer Ther 2006;5:2886–2894.

79 Mengesha A, et al: Potential and limitations of bacterial-mediated cancer therapy. Front Biosci 2007;12:3880–3891.

80 Gorski DH, et al: Potentiation of the antitumor effect of ionizing radiation by brief concomitant exposures to angiostatin. Cancer Res 1998;58:5686–5689.

81 Hess C, et al: Effect of VEGF receptor inhibitor PTK787/ZK222584 [correction of ZK222548] combined with ionizing radiation on endothelial cells and tumour growth. Br J Cancer 2001;85:2010–2016.

82 Mauceri HJ, et al: Combined effects of angiostatin and ionizing radiation in antitumour therapy. Nature 1998;394:287–291.

83 Teicher BA, et al: Influence of an anti-angiogenic treatment on 9L gliosarcoma: oxygenation and response to cytotoxic therapy. Int J Cancer 1995;61:732–737.

84 Carmeliet P, Jain RK: Principles and mechanisms of vessel normalization for cancer and other angiogenic diseases. Nat Rev Drug Discov 2011;10:417–427.

85 Goel S, Wong AH, Jain RK: Vascular normalization as a therapeutic strategy for malignant and nonmalignant disease. Cold Spring Harb Perspect Med 2012;2:a006486.

86 Kleibeuker EA, Griffioen AW, Verheul HM, Slotman BJ, Thijssen VL: Combining angiogenesis inhibition and radiotherapy: a double-edged sword. Drug Resist Updat 2012;15:173–182.

87 Mazeron R, Anderson B, Supiot S, Paris F, Deutsch E: Current state of knowledge regarding the use of antiangiogenic agents with radiation therapy. Cancer Treat Rev 2011;37:476–486.

88 Batchelor TT, et al: AZD2171, a pan-VEGF receptor tyrosine kinase inhibitor, normalizes tumor vasculature and alleviates edema in glioblastoma patients. Cancer Cell 2007;11:83–95.

89 Dings RP, et al: Scheduling of radiation with angiogenesis inhibitors anginex and Avastin improves therapeutic outcome via vessel normalization. Clin Cancer Res 2007;13:3395–3402.

90 Oehler-Janne C, et al: Hypoxia modulation and radiosensitization by the novel dual EGFR and VEGFR inhibitor AEE788 in spontaneous and related allograft tumor models. Mol Cancer Ther 2007;6:2496–2504.

91 Winkler F, et al: Kinetics of vascular normalization by VEGFR2 blockade governs brain tumor response to radiation: role of oxygenation, angiopoietin-1, and matrix metalloproteinases. Cancer Cell 2004;6:553–563.

92 Fokas E, et al: Dual inhibition of the PI3K/mTOR pathway increases tumor radiosensitivity by normalizing tumor vasculature. Cancer Res 2012;72:239–248.

93 Qayum N, et al: Tumor vascular changes mediated by inhibition of oncogenic signaling. Cancer Res 2009;69:6347–6354.

94 Murata R, Nishimura Y, Hiraoka M: An antiangiogenic agent (TNP-470) inhibited reoxygenation during fractionated radiotherapy of murine mammary carcinoma. Int J Radiat Oncol Biol Phys 1997;37:1107–1113.

95 Riesterer O, et al: Ionizing radiation antagonizes tumor hypoxia induced by antiangiogenic treatment. Clin Cancer Res 2006;12:3518–3524.

96 Matsumoto S, et al: Antiangiogenic agent sunitinib transiently increases tumor oxygenation and suppresses cycling hypoxia. Cancer Res 2011;71:6350–6359.

97 Riesterer O, et al: Ionizing radiation and inhibition of angiogenesis in a spontaneous mammary carcinoma and in a syngenic heterotopic allograft tumor model: a comparative study. Radiat Oncol (London) 2011;6:66.

98 Wachsberger PR, et al: Effect of the tumor vascular-damaging agent, ZD6126, on the radioresponse of U87 glioblastoma. Clin Cancer Res 2005;11:835–842.

99 Zips D, et al: Experimental study on different combination schedules of VEGF-receptor inhibitor PTK787/ZK222584 and fractionated irradiation. Anticancer Res 2003;23:3869–3876.

100 Hlushchuk R, et al: Tumor recovery by angiogenic switch from sprouting to intussusceptive angiogenesis after treatment with PTK787/ZK222584 or ionizing radiation. Am J Pathol 2008;173:1173–1185.

101 Kioi M, et al: Inhibition of vasculogenesis, but not angiogenesis, prevents the recurrence of glioblastoma after irradiation in mice. J Clin Invest 2010;120: 694–705.

102 Albert JM, et al: Integrin $\alpha_v\beta_3$ antagonist Cilengitide enhances efficacy of radiotherapy in endothelial cell and non-small-cell lung cancer models. Int J Radiat Oncol Biol Phys 2006;65: 1536–1543.

103 Cuneo KC, et al: SRC family kinase inhibitor SU6656 enhances antiangiogenic effect of irradiation. Int J Radiat Oncol Biol Phys 2006;64:1197–1203.

104 Truman JP, et al: Endothelial membrane remodeling is obligate for antiangiogenic radiosensitization during tumor radiosurgery. PloS One 2010; 5:e12310.

105 Janssens GO, et al: Accelerated radiotherapy with carbogen and nicotinamide for laryngeal cancer: results of a phase III randomized trial. J Clin Oncol 2012;30:1777–1783.

106 Kaanders JH, Bussink J, van der Kogel AJ: ARCON: a novel biology-based approach in radiotherapy. Lancet Oncol 2002;3:728–737.

107 Peters L, Rischin D: Elusive goal of targeting tumor hypoxia for therapeutic gain. J Clin Oncol 2012;30:1741–1743.

108 Belenkov AI, et al: Erythropoietin induces cancer cell resistance to ionizing radiation and to cisplatin. Mol Cancer Ther 2004;3:1525–1532.

109 Machtay M, et al: Radiotherapy with or without erythropoietin for anemic patients with head and neck cancer: a randomized trial of the Radiation Therapy Oncology Group (RTOG 99-03). Int J Radiat Oncol Biol Phys 2007; 69:1008–1017.

110 Wu Y, et al: Endostar combined with radiotherapy increases radiation sensitivity by decreasing the expression of TGF-β1, HIF-1α and bFGF. Exp Ther Med 2014;7:911–916.

111 Ling Y, et al: Endostar, a novel recombinant human endostatin, exerts antiangiogenic effect via blocking VEGF-induced tyrosine phosphorylation of KDR/Flk-1 of endothelial cells. Biochem Biophys Res Commun 2007;361: 79–84.

112 Burrell K, Singh S, Jalali S, Hill RP, Zadeh G: VEGF regulates region-specific localization of perivascular bone marrow-derived cells in glioblastoma. Cancer Res 2014;74:3727–3739.

113 Rios A, et al: Durable response of glioblastoma to adjuvant therapy consisting of temozolomide and a weekly dose of AMD3100 (plerixafor), a CXCR4 inhibitor, together with lapatinib, metformin and niacinamide. Oncoscience 2016;3:156–163.

114 Ahn GO, Brown JM: Matrix metalloproteinase-9 is required for tumor vasculogenesis but not for angiogenesis: role of bone marrow-derived myelomonocytic cells. Cancer Cell 2008;13: 193–205.

115 Danhier P, et al: Optimization of tumor radiotherapy with modulators of cell metabolism: toward clinical applications. Semin Radiat Oncol 2013;23: 262–272.

116 Diepart C, et al: Arsenic trioxide treatment decreases the oxygen consumption rate of tumor cells and radiosensitizes solid tumors. Cancer Res 2012;72: 482–490.

117 Tian J, et al: Darinaparsin: solid tumor hypoxic cytotoxin and radiosensitizer. Clin Cancer Res 2012;18:3366–3376.

118 Sonveaux P, et al: Targeting the lactate transporter MCT1 in endothelial cells inhibits lactate-induced HIF-1 activation and tumor angiogenesis. PloS One 2012;7:e33418.

119 De Bacco F, et al: Induction of MET by ionizing radiation and its role in radioresistance and invasive growth of cancer. J Natl Cancer Inst 2011;103, 645–661.

120 Cokgor I, et al: Phase I trial results of iodine-131-labeled antitenascin monoclonal antibody 81C6 treatment of patients with newly diagnosed malignant gliomas. J Clin Oncol 2000;18:3862–3872.

121 Reardon DA, et al: Phase II trial of murine ^{131}I-labeled antitenascin monoclonal antibody 81C6 administered into surgically created resection cavities of patients with newly diagnosed malignant gliomas. J Clin Oncol 2002;20: 1389–1397.

Martin Pruschy
Department Radiation Oncology, University Hospital Zurich
Raemistrasse 100
CH–8091 Zurich (Switzerland)
E-Mail martin.pruschy@usz.ch

Guckenberger M, Combs SE, Zips D (eds): Advances in Radiotherapy.
Prog Tumor Res. Basel, Karger, 2018, vol 44, pp 41–47 (DOI: 10.1159/000486987)

Imaging for Target Volume Definition and Response Assessment in Lung Cancer

Dirk De Ruysscher · Wouter van Elmpt

Department of Radiation Oncology (MAASTRO), GROW – School for Oncology and Developmental Biology, Maastricht University Medical Center, Maastricht, The Netherlands

Abstract

Target volume definition is of obvious importance in successful radiotherapy. Single-energy CT scans remain the standard, but FDG-PET-CT scans aid the determination of which lymph nodes should be included in the gross tumor volume and to fine-tune areas of cancer involvement. FDG-PET-CT imaging remains the gold standard in clinical practice. Hypoxia and proliferation tracers are still investigational, as is PET-guided redistribution of the radiation dose within the tumor. Contrast-enhanced CT as well as 4D CT scans contain information such as the characteristics of the lungs that are related to individual radiosensitivity, ventilation, and perfusion. Dual-energy CT imaging holds promise for the future for characterization of both tumor and normal tissues. The assessment of response after radiotherapy on the basis of CT scans remains difficult because of inflammatory and fibrotic changes. RECIST is still the standard. FDG avidity suffers from too high rates of false positive and false negative signals and is therefore not recommended, except on clinical indication. © 2018 S. Karger AG, Basel

The definition of target volume is of obvious importance as it directly determines the chances of success in radiotherapy. Indeed, missing part of the tumor will directly impair the probability of obtaining tumor control, whereas defining its volume as too large will result in unnecessary exposure of organs at risk (OAR) to radiation injury. At the same time, a strict definition of OAR is as important as that of the tumor to get the optimal therapeutic ratio.

With the revolution in medical imaging over recent decades, the accuracy of target volume definition has improved dramatically. This has had a clear impact on daily practice, and many studies with the same imaging modality at first glance should be reinterpreted with current knowledge of sensitivity and specificity.

Anatomical imaging with CT and MRI is still the working horse to define the tumor and OAR [1]. However, metabolic and functional imaging done with MRI or PET-CT scans have been increasingly used for radiotherapy planning purposes [2]. In many cases, the heterogeneity within a tumor or inside an OAR has been depicted and quantified aiming at delivering higher doses to more resistant parts of the cancer or to avoid nonfunctional or susceptible areas of an OAR [3]. At present, this remains an area of intense research that has not resulted in practice changes.

Information of metabolic imaging has been shown to improve the standard CT-based tumor definition [1]. It is clear that the boundary between anatomical, metabolic, and functional imaging will increasingly become opaque.

Response assessment has historically relied on volume changes of a tumor. However, it would be of clinical interest to know before volume changes occur if a tumor responds to therapy. Particularly after radiotherapy, inflammation and fibrosis obscure the volume of residual tumor or may even mimic a recurrence. This is where MRI and PET imaging play an increasingly recognized role in patients for which salvage therapy is available.

Here, we will give examples of how the integration of imaging modalities leads to improved target volume definition, with a focus on non-small-cell lung cancer (NSCLC). Not only is the definition of the gross tumor volume (GTV) discussed, but also the role imaging plays for improved definition of the clinical target volume (CTV), although this is by definition not visible. Finally, imaging for response assessment will be discussed.

Definition of GTV in Lung Cancer

At first glance, a CT scan will visualize a primary lung cancer accurately. This seems logical, as the lungs versus the tumor has a high natural imaging contrast difference. However, respiratory movement will induce artifacts in the images, which will decrease the visibility and hence the accuracy of the GTV definition. Moreover, the window/level Hounsfield unit setting and the acquisition parameters of the CT scan have a huge impact on the delineated volume [1]. On a mediastinal window setting, the solid component of a tumor is visible, whereas on a lung window setting small extensions can be detected as well as adjacent ground glass opacities. However, in studies comparing the tumor volume on CT scan with pathology specimens from resection, the tumor as assessed on lung window is larger than in reality. Except for nodules below 2–3 cm in diameter where the differences between CT and pathology are negligible, the CT overestimates the GTV on average by about 5 mm [4]. These are average figures, and a dependency on histology and other characteristics of the tumor is likely. It was therefore suggested that the primary tumor should be defined on the mediastinal setting, but this was based on a small 10-patient study [5]. However, the consistency of the results strongly supports further research in this area.

FDG-PET-CT scanning is the single most important staging examination except for the brain. The long acquisition times of PET scans (order of minutes) compared to respiratory movements leads to somewhat blurred images and a suboptimal resolution, which has led to them being viewed as suboptimal for GTV definition [2]. However, when comparing FDG-PET-defined GTVs to CT and pathology, PET volumes are nearly superimposable to pathology [4]. This is contra-intuitive because the visible CT mass is felt to represent the real tumor mass even if it has been shown that this is too large. Further research, preferentially with 4D-PET-CT scans, is needed [6].

FDG-PET-CT has consistently been shown to decrease the inter- and intraobserver variability to delineate the primary lung tumor and the hilar and mediastinal lymph nodes [1]. The effect is most pronounced in areas with atelectasis. 4D-PET-CT scans could further decrease this variability [6].

Indirectly related to target volume definition is the use of FDG-PET-CT scans for detecting lymph node involvement in NSCLC. As its false negative rate is about 10%, selective nodal irradiation has become standard practice, even in the present era where endoscopic techniques such as EBUS (endobronchial ultrasound) and EUS (endo-esophageal ultrasound) are available [1, 7].

MRI is clearly superior to CT for tumors in the brain or in the pelvic region, but not in the lungs or the mediastinum. An exception is in cases with invasion of the chest wall or the brachial plexus, where MRI is superior to CT [1].

Definition of the CTV in Lung Cancer

By definition, the CTV is not visible. However, it is clear that the microscopic extensions of primary lung cancer are dependent on tumor characteristics and on anatomical barriers. The former has been investigated on CT and FDG-PET scans. It appears that tumors that have a denser outer rim are more prone to extensive microscopic extensions as well as adenocarcinomas [8]. Specific histologic subtypes such as adenocarcinoma with a lepidic growth pattern that is characterized by ground-glass opacities on CT often show a very distant microscopic spread from the primary tumor [9].

The microscopic tumor spread correlates best with CT imaging [4]. In larger tumors, on average, the gross tumor mass as visible on CT scan is actually depicting the CTV and not the GTV. For smaller tumors, probably less than 3 cm, the CT correlates better with the GTV. In practice, a margin for the CTV of approximately 5 mm around the GTV as defined on CT in the lung window, is still considered the standard of care [1]. This extension may be edited according to anatomical boundaries for microscopic spread such as the bones or the large blood vessels [1].

Emerging Applications of Imaging

Intratumor heterogeneity is a phenomenon that has received much attention in recent years. It is known that most solid tumors have a large intratumor heterogeneity (Fig. 1) [10]. These tumors are frequently more resistant to therapy, either chemo- or radiotherapy, and patients have a worse prognosis. Much research has been performed to quantify the various sources of heterogeneity from a biologically or hypothesis-driven approach, for

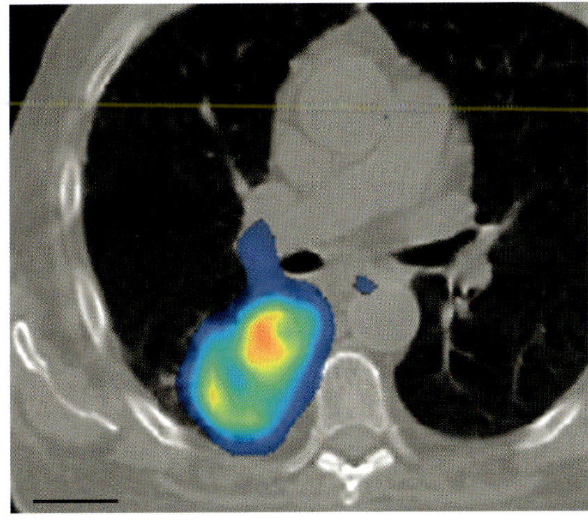

Fig. 1. Clear intratumor heterogeneity on FDG-PET-CT scan in a patient with an adenocarcinoma of the right lower lobe. The red areas depict the most avid FDG-uptake areas, and the blue zones the least avid. Note that in this case, the most avid area is not at the rim of the tumor.

example imaging of tumor hypoxia using hypoxia PET tracers [11], vasculature characterization using dynamic contrast-enhanced CT [12] or diffusion-weighted MRI [13], or imaging of proliferation using FLT-PET tracers [14, 15].

Hypoxia PET imaging can be performed using a variety of tracers currently available which are most frequently based on nitroimidazole (e.g., FMISO, FAZA, HX4, EF5) [11]. Recent studies (e.g., test-retest studies) have shown that these tracers have a spatial and absolute reproducibility. Differences between imaging scans are typically lower than 20%, making them suitable for baseline assessment of hypoxia in solid tumors [16] or for response assessment studies using hypoxia-modifying drugs [17]. In head and neck cancer, hypoxia after the second week of treatment measured by FMISO-PET may serve as a biomarker for the selection of patients at high risk of locoregional recurrence after chemo-radiotherapy [18].

Another attractive imaging modality is the visualization of tumor vasculature. Both perfusion or dynamic contrast-enhanced CT/MRI or diffusion-weighted MRI are techniques that identify surrogates that relate to the tumor vasculature [12, 13]. DCE-CT or MRI imaging allows the quantification and monitoring of changes in blood flow and volume and the permeability of tumors. In lung cancer, these techniques have not yet been routinely introduced in the clinic and are frequently used in a clinical trial setting to monitor for example antiangiogenic effects of (antiangiogenic) drugs and radiation-drug combinations.

The same is true for the imaging of proliferation using FLT-PET. Although some literature shows that there is an advantage of adding an FLT-PET acquisition to increase the specificity compared to FDG-PET imaging [19, 20], this is still not ready for large-scale implementation. Furthermore, the majority of these investigations only involved a limited number of patients (approx. 20–60) for various purposes of segmentation of active tumor volumes [20] or response assessment settings [15].

Another approach to quantifying tumor heterogeneity uses advanced textural features that are extracted from standard CT imaging – so-called radiomics. Radiomics-extracted tumor parameters have been shown to be able to predict 2-year overall survival in NSCLC [21]. Furthermore, these radiomic features are also hypothesized to discriminate between different types of mutations in lung cancer, e.g., EGRF, KRAS, ALK [22]. Defining the most appropriate image analysis and imaging methodology still needs to be defined for these advanced radiomic imaging analysis methods [23]. Radiomics also need standardization in order to ensure reproducibility. One of the major questions to be answered in future research is the relation of radiomic features to the underlying biology. These extracted prognostic features could then also become predictive features and may drive therapeutic decisions and interventions.

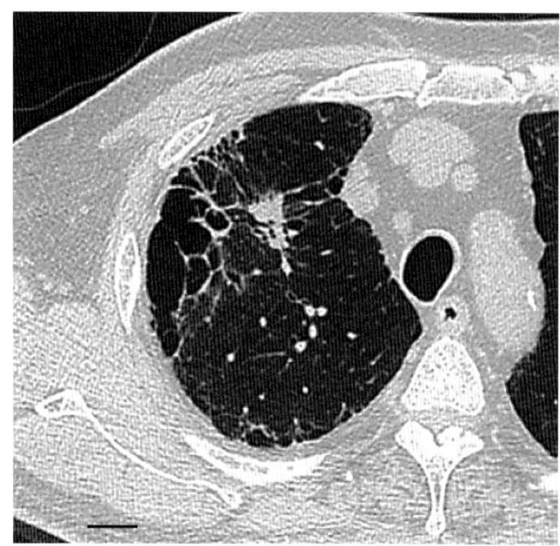

Fig. 2. NSCLC in the right upper lobe surrounded by severe lung emphysema, illustrating the heterogeneity within the lung with zones of fibrosis and nonfunctional air pockets with impaired ventilation and perfusion.

Heterogeneity in the Normal Tissues

Normal tissues are not always homogeneous either in appearance or in function (Fig. 2). For lung cancer patients, differences in regional lung function are frequently present, often due to smoking. It was shown using SPECT/CT ventilation/perfusion imaging that various regions inside the lung typically show differences in function. With the introduction of dual-energy CT imaging and contrast-enhanced imaging, visualization of perfused lung parenchyma is possible. In a research setting, the ventilation component of the gas exchange in the lungs may also be visualized using an exogenous contrast agent such as krypton [24] or xenon [25].

FDG-PET imaging allows for visualization of regions inside the lung that already suffer from a baseline inflammation. Irradiation through these regions has been shown to result in more dyspnea during radiotherapy compared to regions without such a baseline status [26–28].

On the basis of standard CT images, it is clear that the lungs between individuals look different, and also within the same lung important heterogeneity exists [29]. This is to a large extend due to emphysema, a condition that occurs very often in lung cancer patients because of smoking habits. CT defines areas of bullae, i.e., nonfunctional air pockets. On the basis of density changes on CT scans, individual radiosensitivity can be quantified, and the influence of drugs that may affect the tolerance of the lungs for radiotherapy can be quantified [29, 30]. Moreover, CT information allows prediction of the likelihood that a patient will develop infiltrations in a given area of the lungs or between individual patients. In the future, this may help to define prognostic groups with different probabilities for developing radiation-induced pneumonitis, and may aid the redistribution of radiotherapy in the lungs.

Response Assessment

Response assessments have mostly been performed using CT scans according to RECIST criteria. However, as volume changes of the tumor only occur with a delay, and after radiotherapy a mass persists in most patients, there has been growing interest in response assessment with molecular imaging. Contrary to intuition, early volume reduction during radiotherapy was associated with a worse survival [31]. The majority of studies have been performed with FDG as a tracer and most series are small and retrospective. In a prospective study, van Elmpt et al. [32] showed that the decrease of FDG during the second week of chemotherapy and radiotherapy was predictive for long-term survival. In contrast, early FDG changes during radiotherapy alone did not correlate with survival [33]. The clear predictive value of FDG changes early during chemo-radiotherapy was consistently found in many prospective studies [34–36]. For pathological complete remission, the false-negative rate varied between 13 and 25%, and the false-positive value between 19 and 33% [37, 38].

For overall survival, most studies [36–38], but not all [32], did not find a correlation between FDG changes. This may be due to the exact timing of the PET scan at the point at which it is least influenced by treatment-induced inflammation. FDG avidity 2–3 months after the end of chemoradiotherapy was correlated with survival [39, 40], but the therapeutic consequence of these findings is unclear.

In an analysis of the ESPATUE randomized phase III trial, Pöttgen et al. [36] observed that the FDG uptake during the third week of concurrent chemo-radiotherapy correlated with overall survival. This was due to the association of FDG uptake changes and the occurrence of distant metastases, but not with local tumor control. These investigators rightly conclude that intensification of the local therapy on the bases of FDG persistence is likely not beneficial to improving survival, but it may serve as a stratification factor in clinical trials to homogenize the patient groups. Patients showing a bad response may be offered new treatment options directly, such as immune therapy. Other tracers, for example for hypoxia and proliferation, have been investigated and do show a correlation with prognosis, but as the numbers of patients remain small and the therapeutic consequence unclear, this remains even more experimental than response assessment with FDG.

Conclusions

The standard practice for tumor delineation is still CT based, with the aid of FDG-PET-CT imaging and other information, such as endoscopy. Novel PET tracers and functional CT-based imaging holds promise for the future, but prospective studies are needed. Response evaluation is mainly based on volume measurements on CT scans, since the false negative and false positive rates of FDG-PET-CT scans are still too high to be useful in standard care.

References

1 De Ruysscher D, Faivre-Finn C, Moeller D, Nestle U, Hurkmans CW, Le Péchoux C, Belderbos J, Guckenberger M, Senan S; Lung Group and the Radiation Oncology Group of the European Organization for Research and Treatment of Cancer (EORTC): European Organization for Research and Treatment of Cancer (EORTC) recommendations for planning and delivery of high-dose, high precision radiotherapy for lung cancer. Radiother Oncol 2017;124:1–10.

2 Thorwarth D, Beyer T, Boellaard R, de Ruysscher D, Grgic A, Lee JA, Pietrzyk U, Sattler B, Schaefer A, van Elmpt W, Vogel W, Oyen WJ, Nestle U: Integration of FDG-PET/CT into external beam radiation therapy planning: technical aspects and recommendations on methodological approaches. Nuklearmedizin 2012;51:140–153.

3 van Elmpt W, De Ruysscher D, van der Salm A, Lakeman A, van der Stoep J, Emans D, Damen E, Öllers M, Sonke JJ, Belderbos J: The PET-boost randomised phase II dose-escalation trial in non-small cell lung cancer: treatment planning results of the first 20 patients. Radiother Oncol 2012;104:67–71.

4 van Loon J, Siedschlag C, Stroom J, Blauwgeers H, van Suylen RJ, Knegjens J, Rossi M, van Baardwijk A, Boersma L, Klomp H, Vogel W, Burgers S, Gilhuijs K: Microscopic disease extension in three dimensions for non-small-cell lung cancer: development of a prediction model using pathology-validated positron emission tomography and computed tomography features. Int J Radiat Oncol Biol Phys 2012;82:448–456.

5 Wanet M, Lee JA, Weynand B, De Bast M, Poncelet A, Lacroix V, Coche E, Grégoire V, Geets X: Gradient-based delineation of the primary GTV on FDG-PET in non-small cell lung cancer: a comparison with threshold-based approaches, CT and surgical specimens. Radiother Oncol 2011;98:117–125.

6 Chirindel A, Adebahr S, Schuster D, Schimek-Jasch T, Schanne DH, Nemer U, Mix M, Meyer P, Grosu AL, Brunner T, Nestle U: Impact of 4D-[18]FDG-PET/CT imaging on target volume delineation in SBRT patients with central versus peripheral lung tumors. Multi-reader comparative study. Radiother Oncol 2015;115:335–341.

7 Peeters ST, Dooms C, van Baardwijk A, Dingemans AC, Martinussen H, Vansteenkiste J, Decaluwé H, De Leyn P, Yserbyt J, Nackaerts K, De Wever W, Deroose CM, De Ruysscher D: Selective mediastinal node irradiation in non-small cell lung cancer in the IMRT/VMAT era: how to use E(B)US-NA information in addition to PET-CT for delineation? Radiother Oncol 2016;120:273–278.

8 Siedschlag C, Boersma L, van Loon J, Rossi M, van Baardwijk A, Gilhuijs K, Stroom J: The impact of microscopic disease on the tumor control probability in non-small-cell lung cancer. Radiother Oncol 2011;100:344–350.

9 Moon Y, Sung SW, Lee KY, Park JK: Clinicopathological characteristics and prognosis of non-lepidic invasive adenocarcinoma presenting as ground glass opacity nodule. J Thorac Dis 2016;8:2562–2570.

10 van Elmpt W, Zegers CM, Reymen B, Even AJ, Dingemans AM, Oellers M, Wildberger JE, Mottaghy FM, Das M, Troost EG, Lambin P: Multiparametric imaging of patient and tumour heterogeneity in non-small-cell lung cancer: quantification of tumour hypoxia, metabolism and perfusion. Eur J Nucl Med Mol Imaging 2016;43:240–248.

11 Yip C, Blower PJ, Goh V, Landau DB, Cook GJ: Molecular imaging of hypoxia in non-small-cell lung cancer. Eur J Nucl Med Mol Imaging 2015;42:956–976.

12 van Elmpt W, Landry G, Das M, Verhaegen F: Dual energy CT in radiotherapy: current applications and future outlook. Radiother Oncol 2016;119:137–144.

13 Weller A, O'Brien ME, Ahmed M, Popat S, Bhosle J, McDonald F, Yap TA, Du Y, Vlahos I, deSouza NM: Mechanism and non-mechanism based imaging biomarkers for assessing biological response to treatment in non-small cell lung cancer. Eur J Cancer 2016;59:65–78.

14 Szyszko TA, Yip C, Szlosarek P, Goh V, Cook GJ: The role of new PET tracers for lung cancer. Lung Cancer 2016;94:7–14.

15 Everitt SJ, Ball DL, Hicks RJ, Callahan J, Plumridge N, Collins M, Herschtal A, Binns D, Kron T, Schneider M, MacManus M: Differential ^{18}F-FDG and ^{18}F-FLT uptake on serial PET/CT imaging before and during definitive chemoradiation for non-small cell lung cancer. J Nucl Med 2014;55:1069–1074.

16 Zegers CM, van Elmpt W, Szardenings K, Kolb H, Waxman A, Subramaniam RM, Moon DH, Brunetti JC, Srinivas SM, Lambin P, Chien D: Repeatability of hypoxia PET imaging using ^{18}F]HX4 in lung and head and neck cancer patients: a prospective multicenter trial. Eur J Nucl Med Mol Imaging 2015;42:1840–1849.

17 Peeters SG, Zegers CM, Biemans R, Lieuwes NG, van Stiphout RG, Yaromina A, Sun JD, Hart CP, Windhorst AD, van Elmpt W, Dubois LJ, Lambin P: TH-302 in combination with radiotherapy enhances the therapeutic outcome and is associated with pretreatment ^{18}F] HX4 hypoxia PET imaging. Clin Cancer Res 2015;21:2984–2992.

18 Löck S, Perrin R, Seidlitz A, Bandurska-Luque A, Zschaeck S, Zöphel K, Krause M, Steinbach J, Kotzerke J, Zips D, Troost EGC, Baumann M: Residual tumour hypoxia in head-and-neck cancer patients undergoing primary radiochemotherapy, final results of a prospective trial on repeat FMISO-PET imaging. Radiother Oncol 2017;124:533–540.

19 Wang Z, Wang Y, Sui X, Zhang W, Shi R, Zhang Y, Dang Y, Qiao Z, Zhang B, Song W, Jiang J: Performance of FLT-PET for pulmonary lesion diagnosis compared with traditional FDG-PET: a meta-analysis. Eur J Radiol 2015;84:1371–1377.

20 Hoyng LL, Frings V, Hoekstra OS, Kenny LM, Aboagye EO, Boellaard R: Metabolically active tumour volume segmentation from dynamic ^{18}F]FLT PET studies in non-small cell lung cancer. EJNMMI Res 2015;5:26.

21 Aerts HJ, Velazquez ER, Leijenaar RT, Parmar C, Grossmann P, Carvalho S, Bussink J, Monshouwer R, Haibe-Kains B, Rietveld D, Hoebers F, Rietbergen MM, Leemans CR, Dekker A, Quackenbush J, Gillies RJ, Lambin P: Decoding tumour phenotype by noninvasive imaging using a quantitative radiomics approach. Nat Commun 2014;5:4006.

22 Yip SS, Kim J, Coroller T, Parmar C, Rios Velazquez E, Huynh E, Mak R, Aerts HJ: Associations between somatic mutations and metabolic imaging phenotypes in non-small cell lung cancer. J Nucl Med 2016;58:569–576.

23 Yip SS, Aerts HJ: Applications and limitations of radiomics. Phys Med Biol 2016;61:R150–R166.

24 Hachulla AL, Pontana F, Wemeau-Stervinou L, Khung S, Faivre JB, Wallaert B, Cazaubon JF, Duhamel A, Perez T, Devos P, Remy J, Remy-Jardin M: Krypton ventilation imaging using dual-energy CT in chronic obstructive pulmonary disease patients: initial experience. Radiology 2012;263:253–259.

25 Kong X, Sheng HX, Lu GM, Meinel FG, Dyer KT, Schoepf UJ, Zhang LJ: Xenon-enhanced dual-energy CT lung ventilation imaging: techniques and clinical applications. AJR Am J Roentgenol 2014;202:309–317.

26 Petit SF, van Elmpt WJ, Oberije CJ, Vegt E, Dingemans AM, Lambin P, Dekker AL, De Ruysscher D: [18F]fluorodeoxyglucose uptake patterns in lung before radiotherapy identify areas more susceptible to radiation-induced lung toxicity in non-small-cell lung cancer patients. Int J Radiat Oncol Biol Phys 2011; 81:698–705.

27 McCurdy MR, Castillo R, Martinez J, Al Hallack MN, Lichter J, Zouain N, Guerrero T: [18F]-FDG uptake dose-response correlates with radiation pneumonitis in lung cancer patients. Radiother Oncol 2012;104:52–57.

28 Guerrero T, Johnson V, Hart J, Pan T, Khan M, Luo D, Liao Z, Ajani J, Stevens C, Komaki R: Radiation pneumonitis: local dose versus [18F]-fluorodeoxyglucose uptake response in irradiated lung. Int J Radiat Oncol Biol Phys 2007;68: 1030–1035.

29 Defraene G, van Elmpt W, Crijns W, Slagmolen P, De Ruysscher D: CT characteristics allow identification of patient-specific susceptibility for radiation-induced lung damage. Radiother Oncol 2015;117:29–35.

30 Sharifi H, van Elmpt W, Oberije C, Nalbantov G, Das M, Öllers M, Lambin P, Dingmans AC, De Ruysscher D: Quantification of CT-assessed radiation induced lung damage in lung cancer patients treated with or without chemotherapy and cetuximab. Acta Oncol 2016;55:156–162.

31 Brink C, Bernchou U, Bertelsen A, Hansen O, Schytte T, Bentzen SM: Locoregional control of non-small cell lung cancer in relation to automated early assessment of tumor regression on cone beam computed tomography. Int J Radiat Oncol Biol Phys 2014;89:916–923.

32 van Elmpt W, Ollers M, Dingemans AM, Lambin P, De Ruysscher D: Response assessment using 18F-FDG PET early in the course of radiotherapy correlates with survival in advanced-stage non-small cell lung cancer. J Nucl Med 2012; 53:1514–1520.

33 van Baardwijk A, Bosmans G, Dekker A, van Kroonenburgh M, Boersma L, Wanders S, Ollers M, Houben R, Minken A, Lambin P, De Ruysscher D: Time trends in the maximal uptake of FDG on PET scan during thoracic radiotherapy in relation to metabolic response: a prospective study in locally advanced non-small cell lung cancer patients. Radiother Oncol 2007;82:145–152.

34 Huang W, Fan M, Liu B, Fu Z, Zhou T, Zhang Z, Gong H, Li B: Value of metabolic tumor volume on repeated 18F-FDG PET/CT for early prediction of survival in locally advanced non-small cell lung cancer treated with concurrent chemoradiotherapy. J Nucl Med 2014; 55:1584–1590.

35 Eschmann SM, Friedel G, Paulsen F, Reimold M, Hehr T, Budach W, Langen HJ, Bares R: 18F-FDG PET for assessment of therapy response and preoperative re-evaluation after neoadjuvant radiochemotherapy in stage III non-small cell lung cancer. Eur J Nucl Med Mol Imaging 2007;34:463–471.

36 Pöttgen C, Gauler T, Bellendorf A, Guberina M, Bockisch A, Schwenzer N, Heinzelmann F, Cordes S, Schuler MH, Welter S, Stamatis G, Friedel G, Darwiche K, Jöckel KH, Eberhardt W, Stuschke M: Standardized uptake decrease on [18F]-fluorodeoxyglucose positron emission tomography after neoadjuvant chemotherapy is a prognostic classifier for long-term outcome after multimodality treatment: secondary analysis of a randomized trial for resectable stage IIIA/B non-small-cell lung cancer. J Clin Oncol 2016;34:2526–2533.

37 de Cabanyes Candela S, Detterbeck FC: A systematic review of restaging after induction therapy for stage IIIa lung cancer: prediction of pathologic stage. J Thorac Oncol 2010;5:389–398.

38 Zhang C, Liu J, Tong J, Sun X, Song S, Huang G: 18F-FDG-PET evaluation of pathological tumour response to neoadjuvant therapy in patients with NSCLC. Nucl Med Commun 2013;34:71–77.

39 van Loon J, Grutters J, Wanders R, Boersma L, Oellers M, Dingemans AM, Bootsma G, Geraedts W, Pitz C, Simons J, Fatah SA, Snoep G, Hochstenbag M, Lambin P, De Ruysscher D: Follow-up with 18FDG-PET-CT after radical radiotherapy with or without chemotherapy allows the detection of potentially curable progressive disease in non-small cell lung cancer patients: a prospective study. Eur J Cancer 2009;45:588–595.

40 Machtay M, Duan F, Siegel BA, Snyder BS, Gorelick JJ, Reddin JS, Munden R, Johnson DW, Wilf LH, DeNittis A, Sherwin N, Cho KH, Kim SK, Videtic G, Neumann DR, Komaki R, Macapinlac H, Bradley JD, Alavi A: Prediction of survival by [18F] fluorodeoxyglucose positron emission tomography in patients with locally advanced non-small-cell lung cancer undergoing definitive chemoradiation therapy: results of the ACRIN 6668/RTOG 0235 trial. J Clin Oncol 2013;31:3823–3830.

Prof. Dr. Dirk De Ruysscher
MAASTRO Clinic, GROW Research Institute, Maastricht University
Dr. Tanslaan 12
NL–6229 ET Maastricht (The Netherlands)
E-Mail dirk.deruysscher@maastro.nl

Guckenberger M, Combs SE, Zips D (eds): Advances in Radiotherapy.
Prog Tumor Res. Basel, Karger, 2018, vol 44, pp 48–66 (DOI: 10.1159/000486988)

Advances in Technology and Its Application: Radiotherapy Treatment Planning

Markus Alber

Section of Medical Physics, Department of Radiation Oncology, Heidelberg University Clinic, Heidelberg, Germany

Abstract

Treatment planning for radiotherapy has become unthinkable without computer algorithms for dose optimization. Although the need for optimization algorithms originated from the complexity of treatment delivery technology such as intensity-modulated radiotherapy, volumetric-modulated arc therapy, and robotic stereotactic radiotherapy, the focus has shifted to refining goals and methods of optimization itself. Dose optimization chiefly advances in 3 directions: human interface and automation, compensation of changing patient geometries, and diversification/individualization of radiation dose prescription. Traditionally, dose optimization requires the definition of numerical treatment goals, followed by an interactive trial-and-error process to adjust the correct, patient-specific balance of these goals. Being both operator dependent and time consuming, methods are needed that produce high-quality treatments efficiently, with the long-term objective of autonomous dose optimization. Expedient treatment planning is also key to treatment adaptation to changes in patient geometry. Despite all efforts to image and adapt at treatment time, some residual uncertainties remain and must be compensated via treatment planning. Reformulations of the dose optimization problem are joined with various image-based 4D patient models to ensure treatment robustness against geometric uncertainties. Robust optimization leads to a deviation from customary dose prescription in favour of more predictable dose delivery. The dose distribution can be individualized further by additional functional image information, aiming to guide the dose towards undertreated volumes and away from overtreated ones, also known as dose-painting. Multimodal imaging is increasingly integrated into treatment planning, making it a natural consequence to supplant computed tomography by magnetic resonance imaging to establish MR-based radiotherapy.

Trends in Radiotherapy Treatment Planning

Radiotherapy treatment delivery has seen a tremendous surge in technological sophistication that brought its capabilities close to the limits of the laws of physics. Delivery techniques such as intensity-modulated radiotherapy (IMRT), volumetric-modulated arc therapy (VMAT), and robotic stereotactic radiotherapy (SRT) offer great freedom in shaping dose distributions, and thereby question traditional dose prescription concepts, which had to heed the technological limitations of the past. This new freedom comes at the price that treatments can only be planned by employing optimization software. By virtue of this crucial prerequisite, decisions about the treatment are partially delegated to a computer program. This is both a challenge and a chance.

The development of treatment-optimization solutions has been struggling to devise interfaces that allow users to express treatment goals for tumours and tissues in a succinct and intuitive fashion, order them according to their importance, and aid in finding the correct and patient-specific balance between them. As a consequence, treatment planning required a great deal of training, expertise, and time. Development efforts in this area have been directed at making treatment quality more consistent across populations and institutions [1], at making the dose optimization process more interactive and intuitive [2], and at devising schemes for the automatic prioritization of treatment goals [3]. Each of these developments contributes to a more precise and complete formulation of the mathematical optimization problem as a collection of various, often implicit, treatment goals, which is crucial for delegating a part of the decision-making process to a computer.

Once the foundation of dose optimization is established, treatment planning goals need no longer follow traditional rules, but can be formulated more freely. This affects the definition of volume concepts for planning and the prescription of acceptable/required doses alike. The most prominent objective of research is the target volume, where the dogma of homogeneous dosage was questioned by Ling et al. [4], who coined the term "dose painting." Its clinical implementation has been hampered by many stubborn problems with various functional imaging methods, and treatment planning has to find answers to the fact that functional image information will be less than ideal on a broad clinical scope for the foreseeable future. At the same time, the idea of "dose painting by functional imaging" is being expanded to normal tissues.

The other aspect of the target volume that is put under scrutiny is the concept of safety margins to compensate for geometric uncertainties that can occur during delivery. The common procedure to ensure that the target volume, consisting of the gross tumour volume (GTV) and clinical target volume (CTV), receives the desired dose, requires that a larger volume is irradiated so that the target is not missed in the presence of geometry changes, such as organ motion or patient setup displacements. The means to perform this in practice is the planning target volume (PTV), which is a target volume enlarged by suitable margins, solely created for the purpose of treatment planning and treatment plan evaluation [5]. The term "robustness" is often used to express that the quality of the planned treatment does not suffer under the inevitable uncertainties of treatment deliverability. It is increasingly being noted that the PTV method is not the only means to ensure target dose robustness, and that methods that make better use of the framework of dose optimization can create more robust treatment plans and simultaneously better affect normal tissue sparing. A prerequisite for such robust optimization methods are more detailed patient models that require more image information as input [6, 7].

Image information has always played a major role in radiotherapy treatment planning, with computed tomography (CT) still being the mainstay for dose computation and optimization. Other modalities like magnetic resonance imaging (MRI), positron emission tomography (PET), single-photon emission CT (SPECT), on-board cone-beam CT (CBCT), and ultrasound (US) have all found their way into various aspects of treatment planning and delivery, be it for anatomical delineation, setup control, or functional imaging. The technological basis for integrating multiple imaging modalities into treatment planning is deformable image registration (DIR), which is slowly maturing to a level of reliability that allows unsupervised, automatic deployment. With this basis, MRI with its better anatomical contrast can become an alternative to CT for treatment planning. In particular, once the generation of pseudo-CTs from MRIs for dose computation have been established, MR-based treatment planning will constitute a large step forward for many treatment sites [8, 9].

Standardization, Navigation, Automation

The essence of numerical dose optimization is to express the various aspects of "good quality" of a dose distribution in a mathematical function. Naturally, this is a challenge for many reasons, and it is fair to say that formulating this optimization problem is much harder than solving it numerically. Traditionally, every aspect of a dose distribution that appears desirable is translated into a mathematical expression, termed cost function. These cost functions differ in which traits of the dose distribution they favour or penalize, and so a combination of cost functions can yield a comprehensive set of rules by which the algorithm can find the optimum dose distribution. By convention, the minimum of the composite of the cost functions represents the optimum relative to the chosen set of cost functions – which makes this choice crucial. In this approach, there are 3 central questions that need to be answered for each patient case: Do the cost functions express the desired dose traits correctly? Are all relevant aspects covered? Is the balance between conflicting goals, for example target coverage and organ sparing, set correctly?

The last aspect is the most time consuming in practice, as typically between 5 and 40 different treatment goals need to be weighed against each other, and the correct balance is patient specific due to the different challenges that the patient's anatomy may pose. It is important to notice that the quest is not to find the "most optimum" dose distribution, but to choose from a large number of dose distributions that are all optimum relative to their specific prioritization of treatment goals. Two routes have been taken to approach this issue. Firstly, tools to navigate through the large number of potential dose distributions [2, 10, 11], and secondly, the solution of a sequence of dependent, consecutively more restrictive optimization problems that is populated from a case-specific template [3, 12, 13]. Both approaches do not contribute to the first 2 questions.

What makes a mathematical function well suited for the expression of a therapeutic intent? Evidence for the superior effectiveness of particular cost functions is sparse [14, 15], and so are established models of dose response [16, 17]. Thus, it is difficult to refine the maths of cost functions beyond the current set of more-or-less physical dose quality criteria. However, evidence for the effectiveness of certain treatment techniques does exist. An alternative approach to dose optimization bypasses the above problems with cost functions and draws on the strength of existing experience. Knowledge-based treatment planning aims to extract the essence of previously delivered dose distributions and convert it into statistical models. In a second step, these models are applied to a new patient case to predict the dose distribution which is optimally in keeping with the knowledge base [18, 19]. Arguably, this is not equivalent to optimization in the most literal sense, and rather a way to standardize treatments, but the results may be indistinguishable in practice. These 3 main avenues of development are presented in more detail below.

Solution Space Navigation

Real-life optimization is often faced with the problem that one solution may be preferable in one criterion, while another solution may be inferior in the first, but preferable in a second criterion. The choice between these solutions requires some trade-off between the criteria, which is often hard to establish quantitatively. The presence of multiple, conflicting optimization objectives is the subject of multicriteria optimization, which saw its first application in radiotherapy planning in the work by Monz et al. [2]. Successive refinements of the method led to the implementations in products of RaySearch (Stockholm, Sweden) and Varian (Palo Alto, CA, USA).

In essence, the method combines 3 elements: (1) every solution it presents is Pareto-optimal, meaning that every solution is inferior to another in at least one criterion, and superior in a second criterion; (2) solutions can be generated in real-time, and (3) the trade-off between the multiple criteria is displayed graphically. By means of this software, users can arrive quickly at any point in the solution landscape, which is the collection of all Pareto-optimal dose distributions for the given set of criteria (Fig. 1a, b). Thereby, the effect of a change of one criterion on all others can be assessed interactively, leading to a huge acceleration of the goal-balancing effort. In principle, the same would have been possible with traditional user interfaces, yet their lack of responsiveness and visualization would render the interaction much more cumbersome and failure prone. In practice, this can lead to an improvement of treatment plan quality across a patient cohort [20]. Technically, the method relies on the precomputation of a large number of basic solutions, which can be rapidly interpolated while the user navigates through the solution landscape (Fig. 1c). As a consequence, the system requires some preparation time and presents only approximations of the solutions "between" the base solutions during navigation. An area of intense research is based around the fact that the thus obtained solutions do not constitute final treatment plans for IMRT or VMAT, and need to be converted into one at some loss of quality [21, 22].

The fast navigation through the solution landscape circumvents the need to formulate explicit quantitative trade-offs between incommensurate criteria. The user can converge quickly on a suitable balance, especially if the starting point of the search was far off the mark. However, with an increasing knowledge base, it is possible to devise optimization templates that produce a near-suitable solution right from the start. In this case, quantitative information about the trade-off between conflicting objectives can also be obtained via sensitivity analysis [13, 23]. In the context of dose optimization, the sensitivity information can be calibrated in terms of dose, i.e., a decrease in some normal tissue metric by x Gy will decrease some target metric by y Gy. This kind of information can guide the fine-tuning of solutions, but it is inevitably tied to the usage of constrained optimization, which is the subject discussed below. A product incorporating sensitivity analysis was released by Elekta (Stockholm, Sweden).

Constrained Optimization, Templates, and Automatic Optimisation

Conventional optimization schemes rely on the concept of cost functions, i.e., the correct measurement of the quality of a dose distribution by a mathematical formula. The cost functions become the language in which the quality of a dose distribution is expressed. Customary cost functions are maximum, minimum, and mean dose, dose-volume objectives (not more than x % of the volume shall receive more than y Gy/the volume receiving y Gy and more shall not exceed x %), generalized equivalent uniform dose, or

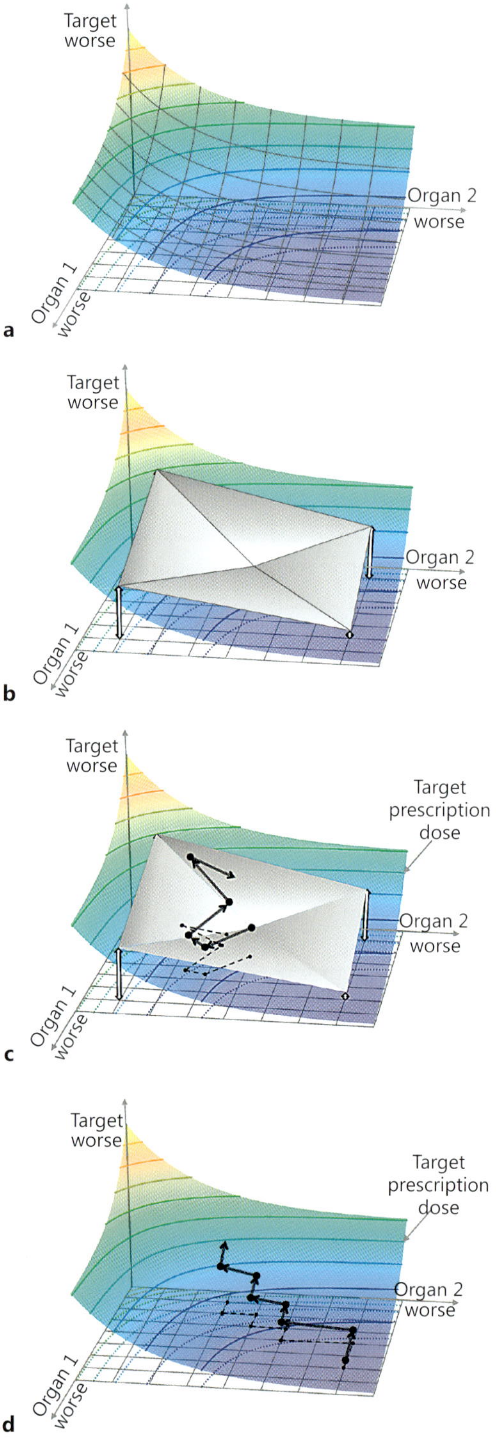

Fig. 1. a Schematic representation of the solution landscape (Pareto surface) of a dose optimization problem. The *x*- and *y*-axes correspond to the cost function values of 2 organs, and the *z*-axis to the cost function of the target. Smaller cost function values mean a better dose. Contour lines represent lines of equal target dose: notice that more sparing of one organ would increase the dose to the other, or reduce the target dose. **b** Approximation of the Pareto surface via linear interpolation of a small number of "anchor" dose distributions, shown as white arrows. Each anchor corresponds to a different weighting of cost functions. **c** Multicriteria optimization: interactive navigation on the approximated Pareto surface presents the user with interpolated dose distributions in real time and offers efficient exploration of the solution landscape. **d** Lexicographic ordering defines the rules on how to progress to a desired solution. A path through the solution landscape can be defined, for example, by repeatedly reducing the cost function of organ 1 while keeping organ 2 constant, followed by reducing the cost function of organ 2 while keeping organ 1 constant, until a predefined target dose is reached. The step-length can be template defined or determined from sensitivity (slope) information.

functions related to these [24, 25]. Recent additions to this set were specialized cost functions to promote generic properties of a "good" dose distribution, like uniformity and conformity of the high-dose region to the target. These already constitute a shift away from the classical organ-based dose prescription and reflect the capabilities of radiotherapy to spare normal tissues to an extent that makes more detailed clinical considerations unnecessary.

A case-specific optimization template would be constructed from a number of volumes that may correspond to organs or auxiliary structures, and a number of cost functions associated with each volume, reflecting the various goals that may apply to the same organ or target [3, 26]. These goals could be prioritized via numerical weight factors, but they are patient specific and hence the template would not necessarily produce a plan close to the desired optimum. Instead, a maximum acceptable value for each cost function could be defined and the optimization algorithm is required to produce a solution that obeys all these constraints. While this does not guarantee that such a solution exists, it would put the solution very close to a fixed location in the solution landscape, independent of the particular patient's anatomy. Modification of the set of constraints would steer the solution to a second, well-defined point, and thereby define a path (Fig. 1d). The capability of constrained optimization to define unique waypoints on a path through the solution space is the basis for some approaches to automatic optimization. In essence, these approaches are concerned with methods for how paths to the desired optimum can be constructed in the language of cost function constraints, and without user interaction.

A direct implementation of this concept was suggested under the name "lexicographic ordering" [3, 12, 13]. It would start with an initial set of constraints and then devise an initial order by which these constraints are tightened consecutively. If the last constraint of the sequence is reached without fulfilling some termination criterion, the algorithm could cycle through the set of constraints again and tighten them further if possible. The path through the solution landscape would be constructed as a sequence of waypoints that differ by only one constraint from their neighbours, with constancy of all other constrained goals guaranteed by the optimization algorithm (Fig. 1d). The sequence of goals, and the amounts by which their constraints are tightened, are defined by the user. The final solution is obtained automatically, and may only require small adjustments, where sensitivity analysis may become helpful [12]. Sensitivity information may also be used to accelerate or partially replace constraint tightening, as implemented in the products by Philips (Eindhoven, The Netherlands) and Elekta.

The efficacy of the scheme was most extensively demonstrated with the experimental software iCycle that interfaces with an Elekta treatment-planning platform [27], and the Philips product [26]. Although this kind of automatic optimization has been shown to generate better results than manual planning in some cases, this should not be seen as a fundamentally superior, different optimization concept – it merely reduces the possibility of human error or carelessness in the planning process. In particular, the traditional optimization interface of cost functions and weight factors does not give an indication about how much of some volume could still be spared without damage to the target dose (i.e., does not provide sensitivity information), which may in practice result in non-Pareto-optimal plans (i.e., some goals could still be improved without deteriorating others). Another fundamental deficit of all cost-function-based approaches, ranging from multicriteria optimization to constraint-based automatic planning, is their reliance on the correct translation of treatment intents into mathematical formulae, which can hardly be taken for granted. Although knowledge-based templates offer a

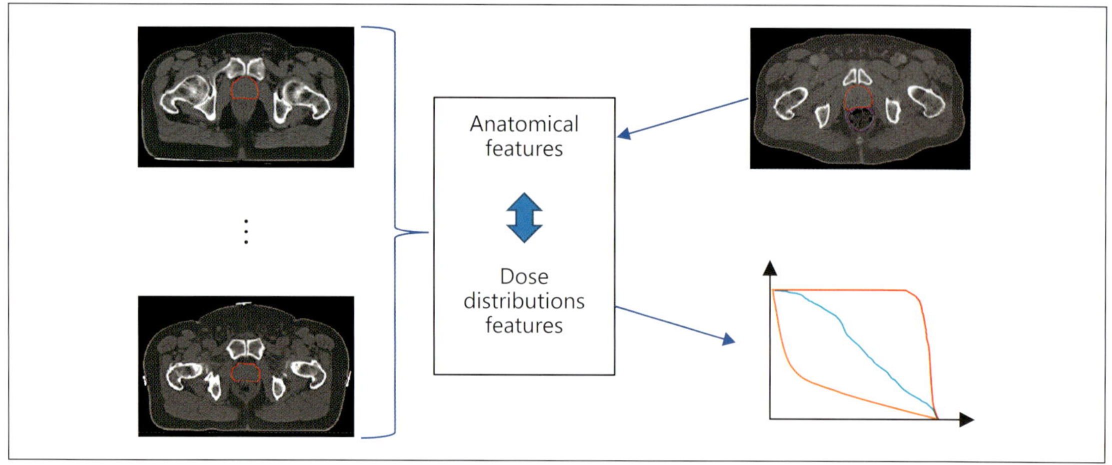

Fig. 2. Schematic representation of knowledge base planning. From a cohort of previously treated patients (left), a statistical model is built that links anatomical features to dose distribution features (centre). A new patient (top left) is first characterized relative to the anatomical model features, and the model predicts the dose distribution that most closely resembles in input cohort.

remedy, the lack of stringency remains a fundamental problem of cost-function-based optimization.

Plan Quality Prediction

Despite all conceptual difficulties, intensity-modulated techniques have been successfully applied to a great number of patients, and both technical and clinical experience has been gathered that has led to a constant improvement of treatment quality. Especially for case classes with a high degree of similarity between individuals, it seems rational to reap the benefits of having ascended the learning curve and find ways to automate treatment planning, not in the sense of optimization, but standardization. Obviously, this starts with an effort to describe the similarities between the anatomic geometries and dose distributions of a case class. The laws of photon physics are quite restrictive when it comes to creating dose gradients within the plane of source rotation for coplanar IMRT and VMAT treatments, and so it is to be expected that general laws can be formulated.

The difficulty was mastered with a combination of geometric concepts, in particular dose-distance maps, and statistical models that can be fitted to the dose distributions of a cohort of previously treated patients [18, 19] (Fig. 2). Any information about the initial optimization setup (cost functions, priority weights) is thereby discarded. The statistical model, once "trained" with cases that cover the breadth of observable patient geometries, can then be used to predict the dose distribution for a new patient. This prediction is then used to formulate a patient-specific optimization template, as described above. The efficacy of this method, in particular the implementation by Varian, has been demonstrated for a number of case classes. Its greatest strength is certainly that it eliminates the human factor and leads to a standardization of treatments [28]. This efficacy can be thwarted by shortcomings of the training data, in particular lack of consistency in the target/organ segmentation, quality of dose distributions, and sample size.

The technologies of automated optimization and plan quality prediction are almost perfectly complimentary. While the former lacks the elements of learning and dealing with cohort variability, the latter has the flexibility of a true optimization that can adopt new evidence and treatment intentions without leaving the knowledge base. The combination of both philosophies are likely to turn out to be very beneficial [29].

Diversification of Dose Prescription

Although the physics of radiation transport dictate that healthy tissue has to be traversed before the radiation energy can be deposited in the tumour, the combination of many angles of incidence (IMRT, robotic SRT) or even continuously rotating radiation sources (VMAT, tomotherapy) and intensity modulation offers a large degree of freedom to distribute the dose. The technical sophistication of photon therapy can even partially offset the physical advantage of particle irradiation with its finite penetration depth. Today, any kind of intensity-modulated therapy could produce dose distributions that are more intricate than are regularly applied clinically. In order to realize this potential, more specific information about the individual patient's anatomy and tumour need to be available. Thus, radiotherapy treatment planning has to include functional imaging modalities like MRI, PET, or SPECT, and also clinical and biological data, into the dose optimization process [30, 31].

Risk-Adaptive Dose Prescription and Clinical Optimization
Given sufficient knowledge about individual tumour and normal tissue biology, treatment planning could directly consider tumour control probabilities (TCP) and normal tissue complication probabilities (NTCP) for individual radiation complications as optimization goals. In practice, both the individual prediction uncertainties and the population-based models for NTCP are too poor for this direct approach [17, 32], rendering biological optimization still unfeasible. Furthermore, more detailed and longer follow-up reveals the extent to which the pathways of radiation complications are still poorly understood, even for life-threatening complications [33]. The mechanics of normal tissue dose response, commonly observed as the volume effect, would determine the formulation of complication-specific cost functions for optimization [34]. In very few instances, it has been reported that a biologically inspired cost function outperformed purely physical parameters in explaining clinical data. Nevertheless, complication and disease control probabilities are the most suitable measure of treatment quality, as no outcome can be sure. The question is then, which elements of NTCP and TCP models can be deployed to treatment planning today with benefit?

Instead of biological models of normal tissue volume effect, dosimetric criteria, predominantly dose-volume constraints that are inferred from clinical data, frequently represent the method of choice. Despite the current popularity of inferring dose-volume constraints from clinical data, there are also severe practical issues with this method [35]. At the same time, it is becoming increasingly clear that clinical and biological cofactors, such as the patient's age, medical history, lifestyle, tumour biology, concurrent drugs, and others, have an equally large influence on the individual NTCP as dosimetric factors. Thus, some means needs to be found to incorporate these factors into dose optimization and trial design [36].

The arguably most elegant approach builds on the mathematics of multivariate logistic regression [37, 38]. Assume some clinical outcome data set was described with a multivariate model, containing one dose variable, v_1. Most of these could be used directly in dose optimization, e.g. maximum dose, mean dose, average dose of the hottest y % of the volume, or volume receiving more than a certain dose (a dose-volume constraint).

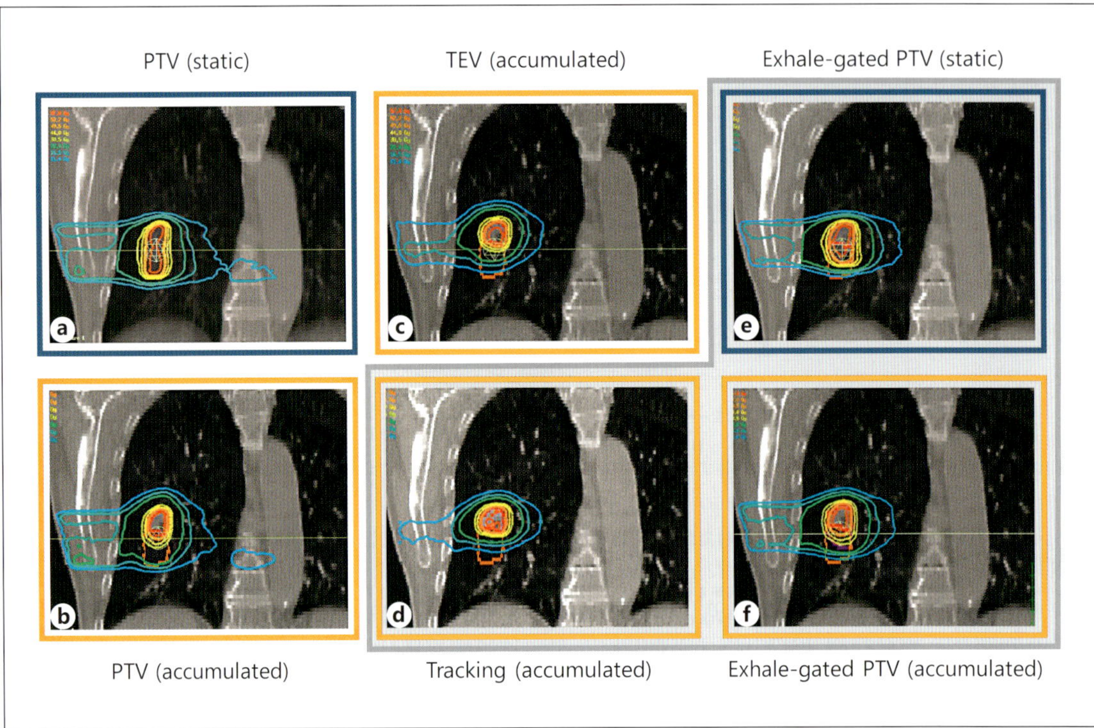

Fig. 4. Various approaches for treating breathing motion during stereotactic body radiation therapy of lung tumours. **a** Classic dose planning on a static patient geometry with an ITV (internal target volume) enclosed by a PTV. **b** Treatment plan of **a** applied to a freely breathing patient results is a distorted dose accumulation in the tissue. **c** Replacing the ITV with the breathing motion information results in an optimization in the tissue-eye-view (TEV). **d** Simulated tumour tracking – the beam follows the breathing motion. **e** classic dose planning for a gated treatment around the maximum exhale phase, planned for the corresponding static geometry. **f** Accumulated dose for gated delivery. Fields in blue frames show the dose computed for a static geometry model of the breathing patient, fields in orange frames show doses in patient anatomy (TEV). Frames with a grey background show the motion-controlled treatment deliveries, and other frames show free-breathing plans. Any kind of motion-sensitive planning or delivery is superior to ITV/PTV planning [76].

surprising result is that the particularities of the prescription function become increasingly irrelevant if the image information is not perfect. For practical levels of sensitivity, the prescription function is already determined primarily by the confidence in the spatial quantitative image information [47]. Thus, while intellectually appealing, the biological modelling required to go from (multi-modal) functional imaging to dose painting by numbers seems dispensable for the next steps of clinical exploration of this approach. The existing data also seem to suggest that pretreat-

ment imaging may be less precise than measuring the initial tumour response to therapy by a second imaging session shortly after therapy initiation. This aspect of guiding the dose painting by treatment effectiveness is extended by Yaromina et al. [53], who suggest including the tumour response to drugs into dose painting treatment planning.

Functional Organ Sparing
Beyond adapting dose constraints to individual clinical factors, it is becoming increasingly recognized that organs should not be seen as homoge-

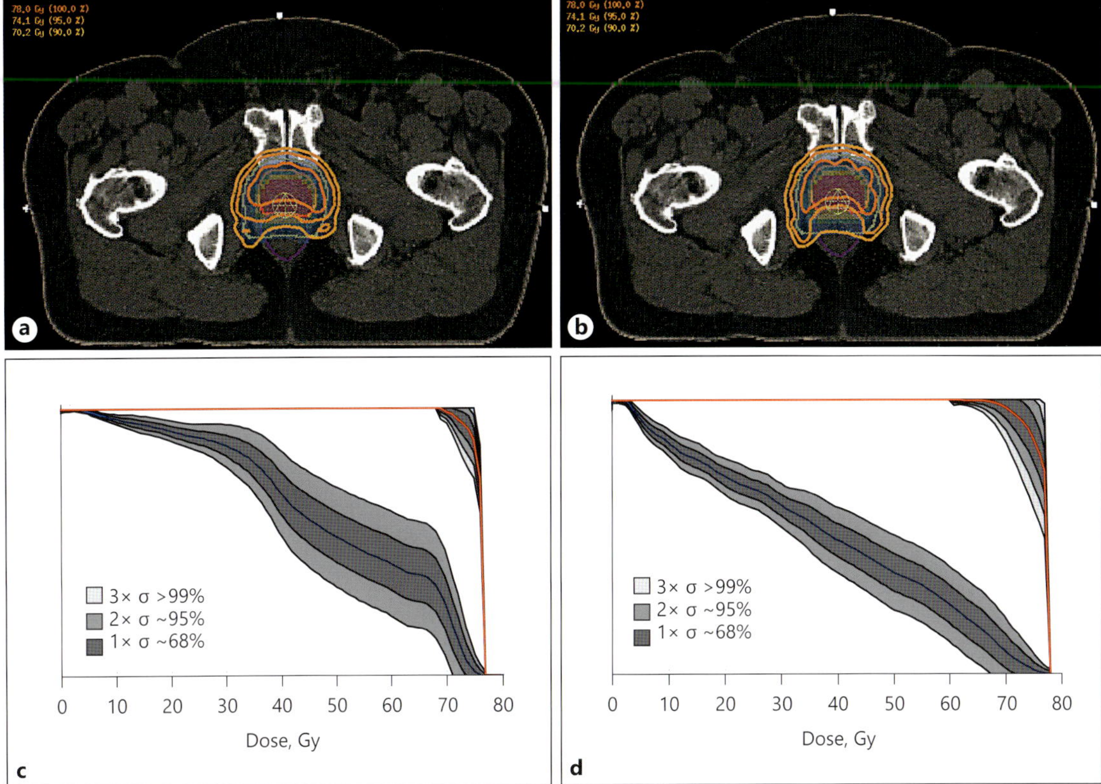

Fig. 5. A prostate case optimized with the traditional PTV concept (**a**) and the coverage probability (CovP) concept [70] (**b**). The heat map overlaid over the prostate shows the probability distribution of finding the target, given organ movement and setup errors. **c** The PTV-optimized dose shows wide confidence intervals for the dose-volume histogram of the rectum (blue) and narrow intervals for the CTV (red), indicating that the treatment is more robust for the latter than for the former. **d** The CovP-optimized dose-volume histograms show more evenly distributed confidence intervals, and a notably better rectum sparing.

neous structures, but as having substructures that are either more radiosensitive or more important for the avoidance of radiation-induced complications. These subvolumes can either be identified anatomically, or via functional imaging. Examples of the former are the hippocampus [54], left atrium [55], or pelvic bone marrow [56]. Although substantial dosimetric improvements were shown in planning studies and deployed to the clinic, direct evidence of reduced complication rates is still rare. Treatment planning to spare anatomical subvolumes usually employs stricter dose-volume constraints than for the entire organ, but does not affect the dose optimization methodology.

In contrast, functional imaging sensitive to perfusion, ventilation, or metabolism [57] can reveal heterogeneity in an organ that is usually the location of the tumour. The hypothesis of functional sparing is the converse of the idea behind dose painting: directing the dose towards subvolumes of low function and away from highly functional volumes could help to preserve organ function [58, 59]. Obviously, this requires that the radiation complication in question has a gradual response, which may be the case for some (e.g., total liver function) and may not be so straight-cut for others (e.g., radiation pneumonitis). The functional information is frequently included by assigning a spatially variable weight to the cost function, i.e., if the cost function is a sum over all volume elements of an organ, each volume element receives a weight that is proportional to the image intensity [58]. Notice that this formulation of a cost function as a sum over all voxels relates closely to the postulation that functional sparing is applied to a gradual dose response complication. In practice, this additional degree of freedom to distribute the dose may have a very variable effect in a cohort of patients, since the defunct areas of lung or liver do not typically align well with beam directions. Direct evidence of its clinical efficacy still needs to be collected.

Treatment of Geometrical Uncertainties

The advent of image-guided radiotherapy (IGRT) by virtue of on-board imaging and lately the development of the MR-Linac dramatically increased awareness about geometrical uncertainties that stem from organ motion, patient setup, or treatment response. A great variety of approaches to compensate for uncertainties have been proposed, but despite all efforts and sophistication, residual uncertainties remain and need to be handled by robust treatment planning. Hence, the basic challenge remains to quantify residual treatment uncertainties. This task constitutes essential quality assurance of any IGRT strategy and requires reliable tools to process the mass of image information: deformable registration, automatic segmentation, dose computation, accumulation, and validation.

Precise information about the uncertainties to be considered is key to not only producing a robust treatment plan, but also to the choice of method best suited for the particular nature of the dominant uncertainties in the given treatment situation. It is neither feasible nor necessary to include all eventualities in robust treatment planning, so a number of schemes with specific usage profiles have been suggested. Efficient processing of image information is essential for all these methods.

From Images to Patient Motion Models
Image information by itself has rather limited use in radiotherapy: it needs to be brought into context and processed. The preparatory stage of treatment planning can be understood as building a model of the patient – traditionally this consists of CT information and volume segmentation. Any data that are collected or generated during treatment planning and application are related to this model: it defines the patient's reference configuration. In this broad picture, it becomes clear that the use of the first CT image set as "planning CT" is a choice honoured by tradition, and by no means unique or superior. Several hard problems in treatment planning were created by a narrow definition of the patient model as "planning CT," and may become solved by moving towards more sophisticated models.

This is particularly true for the twin tasks of DIR and auto-segmentation. Conventional algorithms are centred on the deformation of one image to make it match another. The physical correctness of the resulting deformation vector field is of secondary importance and often enforced by generic rules (e.g., displacement vectors must not cross each other) [60, 61]. In contrast, the algorithms should be centred on the deformation modes of an object, and find the state that most closely matches the image set. The latter is obviously much more laborious, and requires input about the relation of various anatomic structures to each other and their elastic properties. Thus, it is also much more than the common concept of an "atlas," which is barely more than a high-definition anatomical segmentation on a generic image set, unless it is accompanied with some kind of mobility data. Model-based DIR was initially introduced as finite element models for isolated organ systems [62]. Alternatives have been suggested that expand to full body regions and assimilate other methods of treating elastic deformation than finite elements [63]. At the same time, originally model-free DIR methods such as the Demon algorithm, optical flow, or block matching are enhanced by regularization methods that enforce physically sensible vector fields, for example rigid bones, volume conservation, or zero shear. These developments are essential to arrive at a point where DIR can be executed without human supervision, which is an absolute requirement for the management of large amounts of real-time image information [61].

While CT has been the method of choice in radiotherapy for decades because it lends itself so well to dose computation and is readily available, it is by far inferior to MRI when it comes to building and matching anatomical models. To the extent that organ deformation and automated, real-time IGRT workflows become the main concern, MRI outclasses CT for treatment planning. This raises the question of whether CT would be wholly dispensable if synthetic CT data could be created from MRI (also termed pseudo-CT). The main challenge here is the correct identification of bones that have a low signal intensity in MRI, and are therefore hard to delineate with precision. Many suggested approaches resort to the same methods that proved useful for DIR. The solution can also be aided by combining MRI sequences that yield different soft tissue contrast, although this comes at the practical disadvantage of longer imaging sessions. Altogether, many areas of research and technology development are converging towards MRI-based treatment planning that will be accompanied by detailed patient models to handle and integrate the large amount of temporal, anatomical, functional, and biological information that can be put to use in radiotherapy [64, 65].

Real-Time Planning and Quality Assurance

One avenue of research aims to eliminate geometrical uncertainties by real-time adaptation of the treatment to the current patient anatomy. This development is epitomized in the MR-Linac, which is designed to give high-frequency imaging (up to 8 frames per second) during irradiation. These machines would also be suitable for obtaining a full 3D MRI data set for treatment planning at every treatment session. Real-time treatment planning is currently facilitated by porting existing software to special hardware (graphics processing units), whereby the bottleneck lies in the DIR of the planning reference geometry onto the image of the day and the associated translation of the organ and target structures. Some promising approaches exist in research settings [66].

Any kind of IGRT and adaptive therapy is faced with the problem that the dose is deposited in a geometry that differs from the planning reference geometry. In order to accumulate the dose correctly for a fractionated treatment, the dose distribution needs to be warped into the reference geometry, and then added [67, 68]. The same procedure is necessary if intrafractional motion, for example breathing motion, shifts the irradiated geometry relative to the beam. The situation can become even more complicated when the treatment is gated to the motion or tracks the motion. To facilitate this 4D-dose computation, high-quality deformation vector fields are required, which is an impediment for broad clinical deployment. Since the correctly recorded dose plays such a central role, further development in this area is highly relevant.

Another quality assurance issue stems from the fact that real-time adapted treatment plans cannot be validated experimentally, since the patient would have to leave the treatment position. This is in stark contrast to the common practice where dosimetric measurements are the norm. Although devices that record the emitted radiation in front of the patient, or the transmitted radiation behind, are becoming available, they still have to prove their efficacy. Again, the MR-Linac calls for even more radical solutions as the special design of the machines and issues with dosimetry in magnetic fields largely rule out dosimetric measurements. The suggested solution is a second, high-quality dose computation algorithm, which is fed with an adapted treatment plan or the machine status information as recorded during delivery. In order to perform a reasonable quality check, these secondary algorithms need to provide superior quality, which can only be guaranteed by Monte Carlo algorithms or advanced Boltzmann-Equation solvers. Recent developments in software architecture and computer hardware brought the computation times of these algorithms down from hours to a few dozen seconds, which makes them suitable for real-time applications [69].

Robust Optimisation

Another avenue of research is concerned with the compensation of inevitable uncertainties by including them in dose optimization, either by more detailed, 4D patient models, or by reformulating the optimization problem in a fashion that takes the random nature of treatment delivery into account. Even though this seems inferior to real-time treatment plan reoptimization, the latter may not be free from uncertainties either, and often not technically feasible yet. There is a place for robust optimization, especially for particle therapy.

The classical robust treatment planning concept is the PTV, which does work well for the CTV if the chosen margins are large enough. The main criticisms with the PTV are that it may be too conservative in many cases and hence leads to an undue irradiation of normal tissues, and that treatment quality metrics should be based on the dose delivered to the CTV, not the PTV, since the latter is only an auxiliary structure with no anatomical correlate. In order to compute the expected dose to the CTV before the treatment starts, assumptions about the possible geometric scenarios that could occur during the entire fractionated treatment course need to be made. The dose that is actually delivered during the entire treatment course could be recorded by imaging and 4D dose accumulation. Over a cohort of patients, the predicted and the recorded dose should agree on average. Due to the random nature of treatment uncertainties, predictions can never be precise and follow a random distribution themselves. A good set of assumptions about the possible scenarios can at least ensure that the predictions and the realizations have the same random distribution.

Hence, the notion of geometric scenarios and their associated probabilities is central to robust planning. This is already true for the PTV, where margin recipes were derived under scenario assumptions, and even more so for more sophisticated alternatives. Robust optimization concepts can broadly be classified according to 3 criteria: Which uncertainty types do they consider (systematic, random, or periodic geometric uncertainties)? Do they assume dose invariance (does the dose at a point relative to the beam change under the geometry change)? How do they control the random distribution of predicted doses (by its mean, variance, extremes, or shape)? For example, one concept would be tailored to deep-seated targets whose dominant source of uncertainty is organ movement relative to the bony anatomy and would optimize the expected outcome of the target cost functions [70, 71]. This concept would fail for lung tumours that move with breathing motion, since this would invalidate the assumption of dose invariance. These cases might be better served with concepts that optimize the 4D dose distribution, but with customary cost functions [72]. A third concept may be suited for a head-and-neck setting, where some normal tissues need to be spared with very strict dose constraints, which should be obeyed under all circumstances, and where the dominant source of uncertainties are patient setup errors [73, 74].

Regardless of the exact formulation of the concept, they all have in common that they cannot be better in terms of CTV dose than the PTV concept with correctly chosen margins. Some small price in the probability of perfect CTV coverage has to be paid to receive a normal tissue sparing effect, which is usually substantial. The other commonness is the issue that traditional ways of assessing the quality of treatment plans fail – obviously, the dose to the PTV must be worse than it is conventionally, but guidelines demand that the PTV be covered, with no mention of CTV dose coverage. Instead of assessing the quality of a treatment plan by the fictitious dose-volume histogram of the PTV, it would be more meaningful to observe dose-volume histograms of the CTV with confidence intervals. In practice, robust optimization is as much impeded by technical issues as it is by training. To date, there is only one approach that has been applied clinically and was included in a prospective clinical trial [75].

Conclusion

Treatment planning is rapidly moving away from its traditional core – the production of treatment machine parameters and dose computation. The growing complexity on all fronts, be it treatment delivery, imaging, or diversification of treatment concepts, requires an ever-growing degree of sophistication and automation of the treatment planning tools. This evolution is far from over, but it has already overtaken clinical practice on a few fronts, while it is lagging behind in other key applications. The transition towards more automation seems inevitable, but makes it increasingly difficult to assure the quality of treatment planning results. A more holistic view of treatment planning might help to consolidate the advancements of the recent past.

References

1 Li N, Carmona R, Sirak I, Kasaova L, Followill D, Michalski J, Bosch W, Straube W, Mell LK, Moore KL: Highly efficient training, refinement, and validation of a knowledge-based planning quality-control system for radiation therapy clinical trials. Int J Radiat Oncol Biol Phys 2017;97:164–172.

2 Monz M, Küfer KH, Bortfeld TR, Thieke C: Pareto navigation: algorithmic foundation of interactive multi-criteria IMRT planning. Phys Med Biol 2008;53: 985–998.

3 Voet PW, Dirkx ML, Breedveld S, Fransen D, Levendag PC, Heijmen BJ: Toward fully automated multicriterial plan generation: a prospective clinical study. Int J Radiat Oncol Biol Phys 2013;85: 866–872.

4 Ling CC, Humm J, Larson S, Amols H, Fuks Z, Leibel S, Koutcher JA: Towards multidimensional radiotherapy (MD-CRT): biological imaging and biological conformality. Int J Radiat Oncol Biol Phys 2000;47:551–560.

5 Hodapp N: ICRU Report 83: prescribing, recording, and reporting intensity-modulated photon-beam therapy (IMRT) (in German). Strahlenther Onkol 2012;188: 97–99.

6 Birkner M, Yan D, Alber M, Liang J, Nüsslin F: Adapting inverse planning to patient and organ geometrical variation: algorithm and implementation. Med Phys 2003;30:2822–2831.

7 Trofimov A, Rietzel E, Lu HM, Martin B, Jiang S, Chen GT, Bortfeld T: Temporo-spatial IMRT optimization: concepts, implementation and initial results. Phys Med Biol 2005;50:2779–2798.

8 Edmund JM, Nyholm T: A review of substitute CT generation for MRI-only radiation therapy. Radiat Oncol 2017;12: 28.

9 Schmidt MA, Payne GS: Radiotherapy planning using MRI. Phys Med Biol 2015;60:R323–R361.

10 Craft D, Halabi T, Bortfeld T: Exploration of tradeoffs in intensity-modulated radiotherapy. Phys Med Biol 2005;50: 5857–5868.

11 Bokrantz R: Distributed approximation of Pareto surfaces in multicriteria radiation therapy treatment planning. Phys Med Biol 2013;58:3501–3516.

12 Wilkens JJ, Alaly JR, Zakarian K, Thorstad WL, Deasy JO: IMRT treatment planning based on prioritizing prescription goals. Phys Med Biol 2007; 52:1675–1692.

13 Long T, Matuszak M, Feng M, Fraass BA, Ten Haken RK, Romeijn HE: Sensitivity analysis for lexicographic ordering in radiation therapy treatment planning. Med Phys 2012;39:3445–3455.

14 Anderson N, Lawford C, Khoo V, Rolfo M, Joon DL, Wada M: Improved normal tissue sparing in head and neck radiotherapy using biological cost function based-IMRT. Technol Cancer Res Treat 2011;10:575–583.

15 Thomas E, Chapet O, Kessler ML, Lawrence TS, Ten Haken RK: Benefit of using biologic parameters (EUD and NTCP) in IMRT optimization for treatment of intrahepatic tumors. Int J Radiat Oncol Biol Phys 2005;62:571–578.

16 Allen Li X, Alber M, Deasy JO, Jackson A, Ken Jee KW, Marks LB, Martel MK, Mayo C, Moiseenko V, Nahum AE, Niemierko A, Semenenko VA, Yorke ED: The use and QA of biologically related models for treatment planning: short report of the TG-166 of the therapy physics committee of the AAPM. Med Phys 2012;39:1386–1409.

17 Marks LB, Yorke ED, Jackson A, Ten Haken RK, Constine LS, Eisbruch A, Bentzen SM, Nam J, Deasy JO: Use of normal tissue complication probability models in the clinic. Int J Radiat Oncol Biol Phys 2010;76:S10– S19.

18 Appenzoller LM, Michalski JM, Thorstad WL, Mutic S, Moore KL: Predicting dose-volume histograms for organs-at-risk in IMRT planning. Med Phys 2012;39:7446–7461.

19 Shiraishi S, Moore KL: Knowledge-based prediction of three-dimensional dose distributions for external beam radiotherapy. Med Phys 2016;43:378.

20 Kamran SC, Mueller BS, Paetzold P, Dunlap J, Niemierko A, Bortfeld T, Willers H, Craft D: Multi-criteria optimization achieves superior normal tissue sparing in a planning study of intensity-modulated radiation therapy for RTOG 1,308-eligible non-small cell lung cancer patients. Radiother Oncol 2016;118:515–520.

21 Kyroudi A, Petersson K, Ghandour S, Pachoud M, Matzinger O, Ozsahin M, Bourhis J, Bochud F, Moeckli R: Discrepancies between selected Pareto optimal plans and final deliverable plans in radiotherapy multi-criteria optimization. Radiother Oncol 2016;120:346–348.

22 Craft D, Papp D, Unkelbach J: Plan averaging for multicriteria navigation of sliding window IMRT and VMAT. Med Phys 2014;41:021709.

23 Alber M, Birkner M, Nüsslin F: Tools for the analysis of dose optimization. II. Sensitivity analysis. Phys Med Biol 2002;47:N265–N270.

24 Engberg L, Forsgren A, Eriksson K, Hårdemark B: Explicit optimization of plan quality measures in intensity-modulated radiation therapy treatment planning. Med Phys 2017;44:2045–2053.

25 Romeijn HE, Dempsey JF, Li JG: A unifying framework for multi-criteria fluence map optimization models. Phys Med Biol 2004;49:1991–2013.

26 Krayenbuehl J, Norton I, Studer G, Guckenberger M: Evaluation of an automated knowledge based treatment planning system for head and neck. Radiat Oncol 2015;10:226.

27 Buergy D, Sharfo AW, Heijmen BJ, Voet PW, Breedveld S, Wenz F, Lohr F, Stieler F: Fully automated treatment planning of spinal metastases – a comparison to manual planning of volumetric modulated arc therapy for conventionally fractionated irradiation. Radiat Oncol 2017;12:33.

28 Moore KL, Schmidt R, Moiseenko V, Olsen LA, Tan J, Xiao Y, Galvin J, Pugh S, Seider MJ, Dicker AP, Bosch W, Michalski J, Mutic S: Quantifying unnecessary normal tissue complication risks due to suboptimal planning: a secondary study of RTOG 0126. Int J Radiat Oncol Biol Phys 2015;92:228–235.

29 Sharpe MB, Moore KL, Orton CG: Point/counterpoint: within the next ten years treatment planning will become fully automated without the need for human intervention. Med Phys 2014;41:120601.

30 Grau C, Overgaard J, Høyer M, Tanderup K, Lindegaard JC, Muren LP: Biology-guided adaptive radiotherapy (BiGART) is progressing towards clinical reality. Acta Oncol 2015;54:1245–1250.

31 Azria D, Lapierre A, Gourgou S, De Ruysscher D, Colinge J, Lambin P, Brengues M, Ward T, Bentzen SM, Thierens H, Rancati T, Talbot CJ, Vega A, Kerns SL, Andreassen CN, Chang-Claude J, West CML, Gill CM, Rosenstein BS: Data-based radiation oncology: design of clinical trials in the toxicity biomarkers era. Front Oncol 2017;7:83.

32 Deasy JO, Muren LP: Advancing our quantitative understanding of radiotherapy normal tissue morbidity. Acta Oncol 2014;53:577–579.

33 Wang K, Eblan MJ, Deal AM, Lipner M, Zagar TM, Wang Y, Mavroidis P, Lee CB, Jensen BC, Rosenman JG, Socinski MA, Stinchcombe TE, Marks LB: Cardiac toxicity after radiotherapy for stage III non-small-cell lung cancer: pooled analysis of dose-escalation trials delivering 70 to 90 Gy. J Clin Oncol 2017;35:1387–1394.

34 Alber M, Nüsslin F: An objective function for radiation treatment optimization based on local biological measures. Phys Med Biol 1999;44:479–493.

35 Lutz CM, Møller DS, Hoffmann L, Knap MM, Alber M: Reliability of dose volume constraint inference from clinical data. Phys Med Biol 2017;62:3250–3262.

36 De Ruysscher D, Defraene G, Ramaekers BL, Lambin P, Briers E, Stobart H, Ward T, Bentzen SM, Van Staa T, Azria D, Rosenstein B, Kerns S, West C: Optimal design and patient selection for interventional trials using radiogenomic biomarkers: a REQUITE and Radiogenomics consortium statement. Radiother Oncol 2016;121:440–446.

37 Appelt AL, Vogelius IR: A method to adjust radiation dose-response relationships for clinical risk factors. Radiother Oncol 2012;102:352–354.

38 Appelt AL, Vogelius IR, Farr KP, Khalil AA, Bentzen SM: Towards individualized dose constraints: adjusting the QUANTEC radiation pneumonitis model for clinical risk factors. Acta Oncol 2014;53:605–612.

39 Baumann M, Krause M, Overgaard J, Debus J, Bentzen SM, Daartz J, Richter C, Zips D, Bortfeld T: Radiation oncology in the era of precision medicine. Nat Rev Cancer 2016;16:234–249.

40 Lühr A, Löck S, Jakobi A, Stützer K, Bandurska-Luque A, Vogelius IR, Enghardt W, Baumann M, Krause M: Modeling tumor control probability for spatially inhomogeneous risk of failure based on clinical outcome data. Z Med Phys 2017;27:285–299.

41 van der Heide UA, Houweling AC, Groenendaal G, Beets-Tan RG, Lambin P: Functional MRI for radiotherapy dose painting. Magn Reson Imaging 2012;30:1216–1223.

42 Duan C, Kallehauge JF, Bretthorst GL, Tanderup K, Ackerman JJ, Garbow JR: Are complex DCE-MRI models supported by clinical data? Magn Reson Med 2017;77:1329–1339.

43 Boellaard R, Delgado-Bolton R, Oyen WJ, Giammarile F, Tatsch K, Eschner W, Verzijlbergen FJ, Barrington SF, Pike LC, Weber WA, Stroobants S, Delbeke D, Donohoe KJ, Holbrook S, Graham MM, Testanera G, Hoekstra OS, Zijlstra J, Visser E, Hoekstra CJ, Pruim J, Willemsen A, Arends B, Kotzerke J, Bockisch A, Beyer T, Chiti A, Krause BJ: FDG PET/ CT: EANM procedure guidelines for tumour imaging: version 2.0. Eur J Nucl Med Mol Imaging 2015;42:328–354.

44 Kim Y, Tomé WA: On the impact of functional imaging accuracy on selective boosting IMRT. Phys Med 2009;25:12–24.

45 Zips D, Zöphel K, Abolmaali N, Perrin R, Abramyuk A, Haase R, Appold S, Steinbach J, Kotzerke J, Baumann M: Exploratory prospective trial of hypoxia-specific PET imaging during radiochemotherapy in patients with locally advanced head-and-neck cancer. Radiother Oncol 2012;105:21–28.

46 Welz S, Mönnich D, Pfannenberg C, Nikolaou K, Reimold M, La Fougère C, Reischl G, Mauz PS, Paulsen F, Alber M, Belka C, Zips D, Thorwarth D: Prognostic value of dynamic hypoxia PET in head and neck cancer: results from a planned interim analysis of a randomized phase II hypoxia-image guided dose escalation trial. Radiother Oncol 2017; 124:526–532.

47 Petit SF, Aerts HJ, van Loon JG, Offermann C, Houben R, Winkens B, Ollers MC, Lambin P, De Ruysscher D, Dekker AL: Metabolic control probability in tumour subvolumes or how to guide tumour dose redistribution in non-small cell lung cancer (NSCLC): an exploratory clinical study. Radiother Oncol 2009; 91:393–398.

48 Alber M, Thorwarth D: Multi-modality functional image guided dose escalation in the presence of uncertainties. Radiother Oncol 2014;111:354–359.

49 Groenendaal G, Borren A, Moman MR, Monninkhof E, van Diest PJ, Philippens ME, van Vulpen M, van der Heide UA: Pathologic validation of a model based on diffusion-weighted imaging and dynamic contrast-enhanced magnetic resonance imaging for tumor delineation in the prostate peripheral zone. Int J Radiat Oncol Biol Phys 2012;82:537–544.

50 van Schie MA, Steenbergen P, Dinh CV, Ghobadi G, van Houdt PJ, Pos FJ, Heijmink SWTJP, van der Poel HG, Renisch S, Vik T, van der Heide UA: Repeatability of dose painting by numbers treatment planning in prostate cancer radiotherapy based on multiparametric magnetic resonance imaging. Phys Med Biol 2017;62:5575–5588.

51 Thorwarth D, Eschmann SM, Paulsen F, Alber M: Hypoxia dose painting by numbers: a planning study. Int J Radiat Oncol Biol Phys 2007;68:291–300.

52 Jeong J, Setton JS, Lee NY, Oh JH, Deasy JO: Estimate of the impact of FDG-avidity on the dose required for head and neck radiotherapy local control. Radiother Oncol 2014;111:340–347.

53 Yaromina A, Granzier M, Biemans R, Lieuwes N, van Elmpt W, Shakirin G, Dubois L, Lambin P: A novel concept for tumour targeting with radiation: inverse dose-painting or targeting the "low drug uptake volume". Radiother Oncol 2017; 124:513–520.

54 Chamberlain MC: Does hippocampal-avoidance whole-brain radiotherapy for brain metastases meaningfully change current practice? J Clin Oncol 2015;33: 1985.

55 Stam B, Peulen H, Guckenberger M, Mantel F, Hope A, Werner-Wasik M, Belderbos J, Grills I, O'Connell N, Sonke JJ: Dose to heart substructures is associated with non-cancer death after SBRT in stage I-II NSCLC patients. Radiother Oncol 2017;123:370–375.

56 Li N, Noticewala SS, Williamson CW, Shen H, Sirak I, Tarnawski R, Mahantshetty U, Hoh CK, Moore KL, Mell LK: Feasibility of atlas-based active bone marrow sparing intensity modulated radiation therapy for cervical cancer. Radiother Oncol 2017;123:325–330.

57 Partridge M, Yamamoto T, Grau C, Høyer M, Muren LP: Imaging of normal lung, liver and parotid gland function for radiotherapy. Acta Oncol 2010;49: 997–1011.

58 McGuire SM, Zhou S, Marks LB, Dewhirst M, Yin FF, Das SK: A methodology for using SPECT to reduce intensity-modulated radiation therapy (IMRT) dose to functioning lung. Int J Radiat Oncol Biol Phys 2006;66:1543–1552.

59 Farr KP, Kallehauge JF, Møller DS, Khalil AA, Kramer S, Bluhme H, Morsing A, Grau C: Inclusion of functional information from perfusion SPECT improves predictive value of dose-volume parameters in lung toxicity outcome after radiotherapy for non-small cell lung cancer: a prospective study. Radiother Oncol 2015;117:9–16.

60 Sarrut D: Deformable registration for image-guided radiation therapy. Z Med Phys 2006;16:285–297.

61 Brock KK, Mutic S, McNutt TR, Li H, Kessler ML: Use of image registration and fusion algorithms and techniques in radiotherapy: report of the AAPM Radiation Therapy Committee Task Group No. 132. Med Phys 2017;44:e43–e76.

62 Brock KK, Sharpe MB, Dawson LA, Kim SM, Jaffray DA: Accuracy of finite element model-based multi-organ deformable image registration. Med Phys 2005; 32:1647–1659.

63 Teske H, Bartelheimer K, Meis J, Bendl R, Stoiber EM, Giske K: Construction of a biomechanical head and neck motion model as a guide to evaluation of deformable image registration. Phys Med Biol 2017;62:N271–N284.

64 Kupelian P, Sonke JJ: Magnetic resonance-guided adaptive radiotherapy: a solution to the future. Semin Radiat Oncol 2014;24:227–232.

65 Paulson ES, Crijns SP, Keller BM, Wang J, Schmidt MA, Coutts G, van der Heide UA: Consensus opinion on MRI simulation for external beam radiation treatment planning. Radiother Oncol 2016; 121:187–192.

66 Kontaxis C, Bol GH, Stemkens B, Glitzner M, Prins FM, Kerkmeijer LGW, Lagendijk JJW, Raaymakers BW: Towards fast online intrafraction replanning for free-breathing stereotactic body radiation therapy with the MR-linac. Phys Med Biol 2017;62:7233–7248.

67 Ehrbar S, Lang S, Stieb S, Riesterer O, Stark LS, Guckenberger M, Klöck S: Three-dimensional versus four-dimensional dose calculation for volumetric modulated arc therapy of hypofractionated treatments. Z Med Phys 2016;26: 45–53.

68 Heath E, Tessier F, Kawrakow I: Investigation of voxel warping and energy mapping approaches for fast 4D Monte Carlo dose calculations in deformed geometries using VMC++. Phys Med Biol 2011;56:5187–5202.

69 Ziegenhein P, Kozin IN, Kamerling CP, Oelfke U: Towards real-time photon Monte Carlo dose calculation in the cloud. Phys Med Biol 2017;62:4375–4389.

70 Baum C, Alber M, Birkner M, Nüsslin F: Robust treatment planning for intensity modulated radiotherapy of prostate cancer based on coverage probabilities. Radiother Oncol 2006;78:27–35.

71 Witte MG, van der Geer J, Schneider C, Lebesque JV, Alber M, van Herk M: IMRT optimization including random and systematic geometric errors based on the expectation of TCP and NTCP. Med Phys 2007;34:3544–3555.

72 Heath E, Unkelbach J, Oelfke U: Incorporating uncertainties in respiratory motion into 4D treatment plan optimization. Med Phys 2009;36:3059–3071.

73 Fredriksson A, Forsgren A, Hårdemark B: Maximizing the probability of satisfying the clinical goals in radiation therapy treatment planning under setup uncertainty. Med Phys 2015 ;42: 3992–3999.

74 Fredriksson A: A characterization of robust radiation therapy treatment planning methods-from expected value to worst case optimization. Med Phys 2012;39:5169–5181.

75 Ramlov A, Assenholt MS, Jensen MF, Grønborg C, Nout R, Alber M, Fokdal L, Tanderup K, Lindegaard JC: Clinical implementation of coverage probability planning for nodal boosting in locally advanced cervical cancer. Radiother Oncol 2017;123: 158–163.

76 Söhn M, Weinmann M, Alber M: Intensity-modulated radiotherapy optimization in a quasi-periodically deforming patient model. Int J Radiat Oncol Biol Phys 2009;75:906–914.

Markus Alber
Section of Medical Physics, Department of Radiation Oncology
Heidelberg University Clinic
Im Neuenheimer Feld 450, DE–69120 Heidelberg (Germany)
E-Mail markus.alber@med.uni-heidelberg.de

Guckenberger M, Combs SE, Zips D (eds): Advances in Radiotherapy.
Prog Tumor Res. Basel, Karger, 2018, vol 44, pp 67–88 (DOI: 10.1159/000486996)

Stereotactic Body Radiotherapy

Matthias Guckenberger

Department of Radiation Oncology, University Hospital Zurich (USZ), Zurich, Switzerland

Historical Overview and Definition of Stereotactic Body Radiotherapy

In the mid-1990s, the principles and practice of stereotactic body radiotherapy (SBRT) were transferred from cranial stereotactic radiotherapy/radiosurgery by pioneering work at the Karolinska Hospital in Sweden [1] and this concept was quickly adopted and further developed in Japan [2] and Germany [3, 4]. In the next few years, highly promising results of prospective and retrospective studies resulted in the rapid adoption of SBRT for early-stage non-small-cell lung cancer (NSCLC) in the radiotherapy community: a national survey in the USA reported that 57% of all responding physicians practiced SBRT for lung cancer in 2010 [5] and a similar survey in Italy reported SBRT practice in 41% of all responding radiotherapy centers in 2009 [6].

In the beginning, SBRT was mainly defined by a frame-based stereotactic patient setup, which aimed at accurate delivery of conformal dose distributions to extracranial targets. Escalated irradiation doses were delivered in a few or a single treatment fraction, partly because of radiobiological considerations and partly because of the high workload associated with stereotactic patient setup. Today a commonly accepted definition of SBRT does not exist because the frame-based stereotactic patient setup has been replaced by image guidance, which makes the term "stereotactic" misleading (Fig. 1).

A definition of SBRT has been proposed by several national working groups: the AAPM Task Group 101 [7], the American Society for Therapeutic Radiology and Oncology and American College of Radiology (ASTRO & ACR) [8], the Canadian Association of Radiation Oncology – Stereotactic Body Radiotherapy (CARO-SBRT) [9], the National Radiotherapy Implementation Group of the UK [10], and the Working Group Stereotactic Radiotherapy of the German Society for Radiotherapy and Oncology (DEGRO) [11].

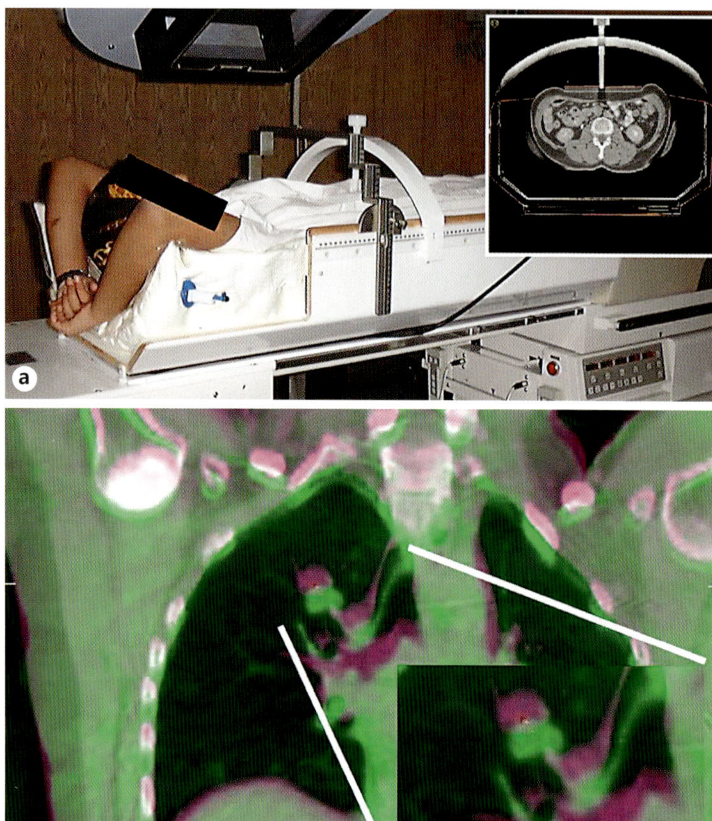

Fig. 1. a Traditional patient setup and immobilization using the stereotactic body frame. **b** Image guidance using cone-beam CT with direct visualization and targeting of the tumor.

Their definition of SBRT all agree on the following items:

SBRT is (1) a method of external beam radiotherapy (EBRT), to (2) accurately deliver a (3) high dose of irradiation in (4) one or few treatment fractions to an (5) extracranial target. These essential components of the SBRT definition are described in more detail below.

1. SBRT can be adequately performed with either traditional linear accelerators equipped with suitable image-guidance technology, linear accelerators specifically adapted for SBRT, and dedicated delivery systems. Additionally, the principles of SBRT apply for both photon and particle therapy.

2. Systemic optimization of the whole workflow and appropriate quality assurance proce-

dures are fundamental in SBRT. Importantly, this includes both the clinical part as well as the technical/physical part of treatment planning and delivery. Therefore, SBRT is a multidisciplinary (all professions involved in lung cancer care) and multiprofessional (radiation oncologists, medical physicists, and radiation technologists) team approach with close collaboration of all partners. Dedicated teaching and training, credentialing and the development of written protocols are essential components of the quality assurance.

3, 4. Irradiation doses, which are at least equivalent to radical doses in conventional fractionation, are delivered in a few fractions or even a single fraction as radiosurgery. From a radiobiological perspective, there is no clearly defined maximum number of treatment fractions for definition of SBRT. In contrast, reimbursement issues explain the limitation to a maximum of 5 SBRT fractions in the USA. Considering current SBRT practice and outcomes, SBRT should be delivered in a maximum of 8–12 fractions but a higher fraction number may be meaningful in certain clinical situations. In general, adjustment of single-fraction dose and total dose to size and location of the target is essential.

5. The target needs to be spatially separated from critical organs at risk (OAR) without diffuse infiltration into them. Only the macroscopic target and small, immediately adjacent volumes of potential microscopic spread are treated in SBRT. This target is accurately localized by daily image guidance using tumor site-specific imaging modalities.

Even if no frame-based patient setup using external stereotactic coordinates is performed, the term "stereotactic" is still considered as appropriate. External stereotactic coordinates are replaced by internal coordinates of the patient's anatomy, which is visualized by image guidance and compared with pretreatment planning images. Image guidance targets the macroscopic soft tissue tumor itself or surrogate anatomical structures/fiducial markers, which are closely correlated to the target.

Stereotactic ablative radiotherapy has been proposed by an international group as an alternative acronym to SBRT [12]. If SBRT is practiced with very high single-fraction doses and total doses, for example 3 fractions of 20 Gy as proposed by McGarry et al. [13], the treatment is certainly ablative by destruction of all tumor and normal tissue within the target volume. However, we are frequently challenged with a situation where critical serial OARs are in very close vicinity to the tumor and physical sparing is impossible. In such situations, fractionation has been shown to spare these OARs while biological effective doses are still sufficiently high

to achieve local tumor control [14]. It is debatable whether such treatments are best described as ablative.

SBRT is today practiced and evaluated in many cancers and many clinical situations and stages. However, the strongest evidence is available for the application in NSCLC. Therefore, the value, benefits, limitations, and challenges of SBRT will be illustrated using NSCLC as an example.

SBRT for Early-Stage NSCLC

If NSCLC is detected at an early stage, surgical treatment with lobectomy and systematic hilar and mediastinal lymph node dissection achieves excellent 5-year overall survival (OS) of 68–92% [15]. Current international guidelines by ESMO and NCCN therefore describe lobectomy as the treatment of choice for patients who are medically and technically operable and accept the risk of the surgical procedure. However, if lung cancer is detected in elderly patients, up to a quarter of the patients remain untreated [16], despite the prognosis of untreated early-stage lung cancer being very poor. Furthermore, the proportion of patients not treated surgically has increased in the USA over recent years. This is most likely the result of more frequent diagnoses of lung cancer in elderly patients with multiple and severe comorbidities, who are at increased surgical risks and have a worse prognosis [17, 18].

For such elderly and fragile patients, an alternative curative treatment option is eagerly awaited: this treatment is ideally noninvasive, associated with low toxicity, and is performed as an outpatient procedure in one or a few sessions.

Until about 20 years ago, conventionally fractionated radiotherapy was the treatment of choice in inoperable patients with early-stage NSCLC. The primary cancer as well as elective lymph nodes were treated with radiation doses of 60–66 Gy delivered in 30–33 fractions. However, this irradiation dose and technique achieved long-term local tumor control in only 60% of the patients, resulting in a poor OS of 40% at 3 years [19]. Despite patients treated with radiotherapy being different to surgical cohorts (older and suffering from more and severe comorbidities), most patients died from lung cancer, and local disease recurrence was the most frequent pattern of failure.

SBRT substantially changed the treatment of early-stage NSCLC compared to the traditional radiotherapy practice, by integration of advanced technologies into staging, radiotherapy planning, and delivery. After FDG-PET nodal staging with a cN0 result, only the primary tumor is treated, notably without elective radiation. Breathing-induced motion of the tumor is assessed on an individual patient level, integrated into target volume definition and radiotherapy delivery: active and passive 4D motion compensation strategies are used, both achieving an excellent and consistent outcome. Highly conformal treatment planning is combined with accurate dose calculation. At the time of treatment delivery, patient immobilization and daily image guidance ensure irradiation of the tumor with millimeter accuracy. All these technologies allow safe delivery of highly escalated irradiation doses beyond 100-Gy BED (biological equivalent dose). A case example is illustrated in Figure 2.

SBRT for Inoperable Patients with Stage I NSCLC
SBRT has been evaluated within 7 prospective phase II clinical trials, where 394 patients were treated altogether [20–26]: evidence for using SBRT in medically inoperable patients is therefore based on a broad evidence level. Detailed results are summarized in Table 1. All clinical trials included patients with early-stage NSCLC, who were judged medically inoperable in interdisciplinary tumor boards. The majority of clinical trials only included patients with histopathologically proven lung cancer; in the remaining 3 clinical trials, biopsy confirmation of disease was made in a minimum of 66% of the patients.

Local tumor control at 2–7 years was consistently >84%, and in 3 out of 7 studies was >90%. The duration of follow-up in the individual studies had no obvious influence on local tumor control: despite late local recurrences having been described after SBRT, the prospective trial with the longest follow-up of a median of 86 months by Sun et al. [26] had excellent local tumor control of 92%.

The most relevant factor influencing the local tumor control after SBRT is the radiation dose. All modeling studies consistently show that a minimum dose of 100-Gy BED is required to achieve long-term local tumor control of a minimum of 90% [27–29]. This is relevant, because a learning curve has been observed regarding this issue. The patterns of care study by the DEGRO working group on stereotactic radiotherapy reported outcomes in 582 stage I NSCLC patients treated at 13 centers between 1998 and 2011. Overall, local tumor control was only 80% at 3 years [30]. However, the SBRT dose had been continuously increased in the first decade of SBRT practice and, as a result, patients treated with a minimum of 106-Gy BED (n = 164) achieved excellent local tumor control of 93%, which is in perfect agreement with results of prospective trials.

Dose response modeling is especially challenging in SBRT because of the large variability in terms of fractionation: SBRT is delivered in single fraction radiosurgery and fractionated radiotherapy with up to 10–12 fractions. Comparison of physical doses and their use for outcome modeling is obviously not meaningful. However, the value and accuracy of the linear-quadratic model (LQ-model) for the calculation of biologically effective doses has been discussed controversially [31]. Recent studies have shown that the LQ-model accurately describes the biological efficacy even in very high-dose SBRT [32];

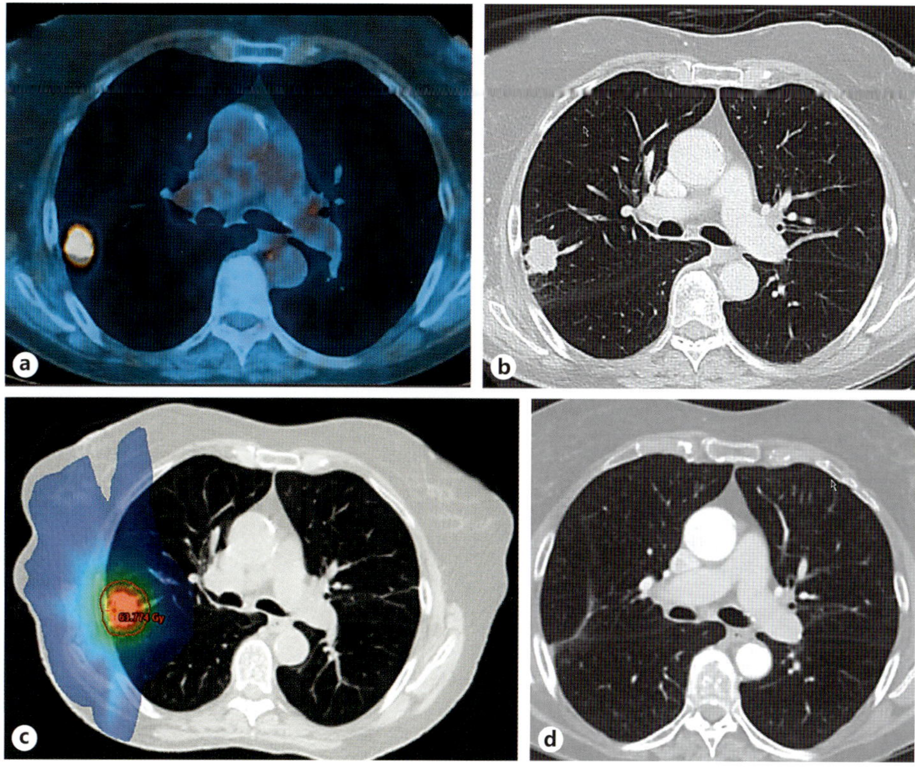

Fig. 2. Case example of a 79-year-old female diagnosed with stage I NSCLC, judged medically inoperable by the multidisciplinary tumor board: FDG-PET CT staging (**a**); diagnostic CT of the thorax (**b**); SBRT with illustration of conformal irradiation doses (**c**), and follow-up CT of the thorax 18 months after SBRT (**d**).

more complex radiobiological models did not achieve improved results compared to the LQ-model [33].

In contrast to consistent results regarding local tumor control, OS at 5 years varies between 30 and 83%. This is best explained by the fact that the majority of patients did not die of lung cancer but of their comorbidities, which had been the reason for their interoperability. The highly significant influence of comorbidities on OS in patients with early-stage NSCLC has been clearly shown after SBRT [34] and surgery [18]. The variability in OS is best explained by inconsistent definitions of "interoperability," and therefore the inclusion of patients with different degrees of comorbidities, and therefore different prognoses. Cancer-specif-

ic survival after SBRT is thus consistently between 73 and 82%.

The pattern of disease-free disease recurrence is distant: between 10 and 20% of patients will develop distant metastases. The most relevant factor for an increased risk of distant metastasis is the size of the primary tumor. Additionally, activity of the primary tumor in FDG-PET [35] and contact of the primary cancer to the pleura [36, 37] were associated with the risk of distant metastasis. Regional recurrences and in hilar or mediastinal lymph nodes are observed in a maximum 10% of the patients following adequate staging using FDG-PET.

SBRT is characterized by a highly favorable toxicity profile. Despite the selection and treatment of high-risk patients with older age suffer-

Table 1. Oncological outcome of SBRT for early-stage NSCLC in prospective trials and large retrospective analyses

Study	Publication year	Patients, n	Histopathological confirmation of malignancy, %	Median follow-up, months	Endpoint assessment	OS	DSS	LC
Prospective phase II studies								
Nagata et al. [20]	2005	45	100	30	5a	72–83%	–	95–100%
Lindberg et al. [25]	2015	57	66	42	5a	30%	74%	79%
Fakiris et al. [21]	2009	70	100	50	3a	43%	82%	88%
Ricardi et al. [22]	2010	62	64	28	3a	57%	73%	88%
Timmerman et al. [23]	2010	55	100	34	3a	56%	–	91%
Bral et al. [24]	2011	40	72	16	2a	52%	–	84%
Sun et al. [26]	2017	65	100	8	7a	48%	–	92%
Overall		394	64–100	16–86		30–83%	73–82%	79–100%
Large retrospective analyses								
Senthi et al. [44]	2012	676	35	33	5a	median 41 months	median not reached	89%
Grills et al. [46]	2012	505	64	19	2a	60%	87%	94%
Guckenberger et al. [30]	2013	582	85	21	3a	47%	–	80%
		164				62%		93%
Zhao et al. [45]	2016	1,092	100	32	5a	45%	–	94%
Overall		2,855	35–100%	19–33		45–60%		80–94%

OS, overall survival.

ing from severe comorbidities, SBRT-related mortality is consistently <1%. Only one study reported a very high SBRT-induced mortality of 7% [21] (Table 2). This worrisome but isolated mortality is explained by 2 factors: the radiation dose was very high in this trial with 3 fractions of 20–22 Gy, and this excessive radiation dose was not only applied in peripherally located lung cancer, but also centrally located tumors [38]. The following part of this chapter will go deeper into this issue of risk-adapted fractionation. Overall, clinically relevant toxicity (grade >II) is observed in <20% of patients, and in 5 out of 7 prospective studies in <10% of patients. Grade IV toxicity has been described only very rarely. The most frequently observed toxicity after high-dose stereotactic radiotherapy is a radiation-induced pneumonitis and dyspnea. The risk of pulmonary toxicity de-

pends on the dose exposure of the lungs and is therefore associated with the size and location of the cancer as well as radiotherapy technique [39]. Very rare toxicities after SBRT are rib fractures, fibrosis, and neuralgia of the chest wall, brachial plexopathy, and vertebral fractures. All of these toxicities can be minimized using modern therapy technologies.

After SBRT with curative intent, quality of life remains stable and unaffected. Conversely, it has been reported that quality of life improves in some subdomains. This was consistently observed in prospective [40] and retrospective [41, 42] studies. Especially pulmonary domains of quality of life are not negatively affected by radiotherapy: objective pulmonary function parameters (FEF1 and DLCO) decrease on average by 5–10% after small volume SBRT [43], and these

Table 2. Toxicity after SBRT for early-stage NSCLC in prospective trials and large retrospective analyses

Study	Publication year	Patients, n	Toxicity >grade II	Mortality, %
Prospective phase II studies				
Nagata et al. [20]	2005	45	0%	0
Lindberg et al. [25]	2015	57	Within 3a – G3: 28%	
			After 3a – G3: 9%	0
Fakiris et al. [21]	2009	70	Peripheral location – G3–5: 10%	
			Central location – G3–5: 27%	7
Ricardi et al. [22]	2010	62	G3: 3%	0
Timmerman et al. [23]	2010	55	G3: 24%	0
			G4: 4%	
Bral et al. [24]	2011	40	Pulmonary toxicity – G3: 20%	0
Sun et al. [26]	2017	65	G3: 4.6%	0
Large retrospective analyses				
Senthi et al. [44]	2012	676	–	–
Grills et al. [46]	2012	505	Radiation-induced pneumonitis – G3: 3%	0.2
Guckenberger et al. [30]	2013	582	Radiation-induced pneumonitis – G2–3: 7.4%	0.4
Zhao et al. [45]	2016	1,092	–	–

small changes are without consequences for patient-reported quality of life.

These excellent results of SBRT were not only reproduced in prospective studies, but also in retrospective studies and patterns of care analyses. Table 1 summarizes the results of SBRT for stage I NSCLC, which were observed outside of prospective clinical trials within daily routine practice. All studies included a minimum of 500 patients, involving 2,855 patients in total. Two studies are large single institutional analyses [44, 45], one study reports outcomes from 5 international centers [46], and the stereotactic study of the DEGRO working group reports patterns of care and patterns of outcome from all 13 centers from German-speaking countries [30]. Local tumor control was consistently >90% if sufficiently high radiation doses were delivered. OS ranged between 45 and 60% after 3–5 years, which is in agreement with prospective trials. SBRT-induced mortality was below 1% in all studies, and toxicity grade ≥3 was observed in <10% of the patients. These data prove that safe and effective practice of the com-

plex SBRT technique outside of prospective clinical trials in daily routine practice is possible. In analogy to surgical experiences, a volume effect was observed for SBRT such that a minimum number of patients treated with SBRT was required for generating sufficient SBRT experience and achieving an optimal outcome [47, 48].

Controversies in SBRT for Early-Stage NSCLC
Despite consistent and promising results of SBRT for early-stage NSCLC, several details of SBRT practice and interpretations of its outcome have been discussed controversially.

The results of SBRT in early-stage NSCLC are sometimes challenged by the fact that histopathological confirmation of disease was not obtained in all patients prior to treatment. It is speculated whether the good results of SBRT may at least in part be the result of treatment of nonmalignant lesions and not of true cancer. Regarding this issue, it should be noted that the majority of the prospective studies obtained histopathological confirmation of malignancy in 100% of the patients [20, 21, 23, 26], and this was also true for the largest single-institution analysis [45]. Overall, there is only one large single-center experience with histopathological confirmation in less than half of the patients [44]: additional analyses from that center clearly showed that the results of patients with and without histopathological confirmation of malignancy are identical [49]. Although a few patients might have been treated with SBRT for nonmalignant lesions, their small number did not have any influence on the overall outcome reported for SBRT. Nevertheless, all national and international guidelines recommend histopathological confirmation prior to SBRT. However, there are patients where this is not possible for technical reasons or where the procedure is considered too risky. In this situation, guidelines do allow SBRT based on the clinical diagnosis of lung cancer.

In SBRT, only the primary tumor is treated without elective nodal irradiation. This is also in agreement with locally advanced lung cancer, where elective treatment of noninvolved lymph node stations is not performed after accurate staging using FDG-PET. In Western European countries with low incidence rates of lung granulomatous diseases, FDG-PET is false negative in only about 10–12% [50, 51]. Whether this accuracy is improved by additional EUS and EBUS staging in FDG-PET cN0 patients is currently being evaluated in prospective clinical trials.

After SBRT, fibrotic changes of the normal tissue in the high-dose region is observed in the majority of patients. This is especially true for the lung. Two clinical examples are shown in Figure 3. The fibrotic changes after SBRT are dose dependent and their morphology changes for years after treatment [52]. Recently, CT-based morphological criteria have been described to differentiate between normal tissue changes and true tumor recurrence. External validation using only 2 CT-based criteria achieved a sensitivity of 92% and specificity of 85% (bulging margin and cranial causal growth) [53]. In cases of uncertain CT findings, follow-up using FDG PET is recommended. However, FDG-PET should not be performed within the first 6 months after SBRT because of inflammatory and FDG-PET-positive normal tissue reactions after the treatment.

High-Risk Situations for SBRT
Excellent results of SBRT regarding safety and efficacy are based on the treatment of lung tumors <5 cm in diameter and with a peripheral location surrounded by lung tissue.

The reasons for SBRT and against surgical resection are pulmonary comorbidities in the majority of patients, especially smoking-associated COPD. It has been shown that SBRT is also safe in patients with severe COPD and a very small pulmonary reserve [54]. This is explained by highly focal irradiation with optimal sparing of the lung, which is a parallel organized critical structure. However, recent studies have described that interstitial lung disease might be a relevant risk factor for SBRT. Several studies reported very high rates of high-grade and even lethal toxicities in the presence of this comorbidity [55–57]. Consequently, we need to be cautious when expanding the indication of SBRT to patient cohorts with rare comorbidities, where interactions may trigger high and unexpected rates of severe toxicity.

SBRT with its main characteristics of a very high radiation dose delivered to small volumes has been proven safe when applied in tumors located within parallel structured organs, such as the lung and liver. However, this favorable toxicity profile may be different if serial OARs are close by to the target or even within the target volume. In pulmonary SBRT, high rates of severe toxicity have been reported when centrally located tumors were treated [38]: a central location was defined as the tumor being within 2 cm of the proximal bronchial tree. Critical OARs in SBRT for centrally located tumors are the esoph-

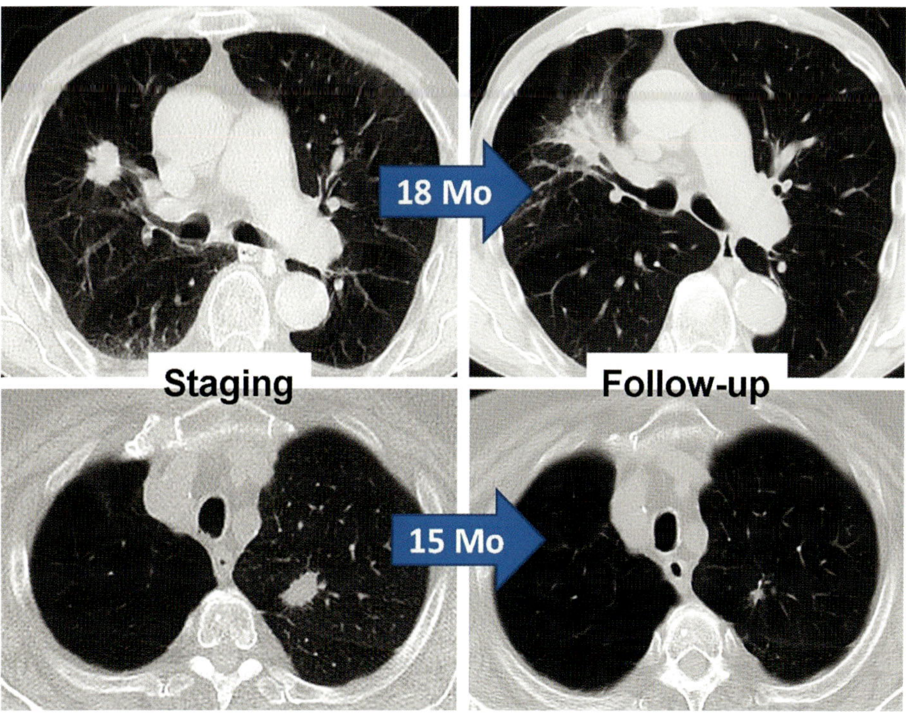

Fig. 3. Case examples of CT-based follow-up after SBRT. Above, fibrotic changes in the high-dose volume; below, minimal fibrotic changes. Mo, months.

agus, central bronchi, trachea, large vessels, and the heart. In the treatment of lower lobe tumors, very high irradiation doses may reach the stomach and bowel; in the treatment of upper lobe tumors, very high irradiation doses may reach the brachial plexus. Best possible sparing of these organs by conformal avoidance is of highest priority. If physical sparing is not sufficient, biological sparing of serial OAR by more fractionated radiotherapy should be performed. This is called risk-adapted fractionation and has become the standard of care to treat centrally located lung tumors [14, 58]. Similar risk-adapted fractionation is also performed for sparing OAR, described above.

The experiences of SBRT are based on the treatment of tumors with diameters <5 cm, mostly between 2 and 3 cm. Treatment of larger tumors always results in increased exposure of nor-mal tissue with a high irradiation dose, and will decrease the technological benefits of SBRT. The experiences of SBRT for tumors larger than 5 cm are based on small retrospective studies: despite toxicity overall appearing to be acceptable, a few studies also reported an increased risk of toxicity [59–61]. Consequently, similar to experience with tumors located close to critical OARs, more fractionated SBRT regimes should be considered when larger tumors are treated.

Finally, experiences of SBRT are mostly based on the treatment of solitary intrapulmonary tumors. This is also true for intrahepatic tumors, where mostly solitary lesions were treated. The treatment of multiple lesions within one organ [62, 63] should therefore be practiced only with caution – dose distributions of all SBRT treatments need to be accumulated to perform a global risk assessment.

Table 3. Overview of SBRT studies

Study	Study type	Patients, n	3a OS, %	5a OS, %
Chang et al. [64], 2015	Pooled analysis of 2 randomized trials	31	95	–
Nagata et al. [65], 2015	Prospective phase II study	64	76.5	54
Uematsu et al. [66], 2001	Retrospective analysis	29	86	–
Lagerwaard et al. [67], 2012	Retrospective analysis	177	84.7	51.3
Grills et al. [46], 2012	Retrospective analysis	56	78[a]	–
Onishi et al. [68], 2011	Retrospective analysis	87	–	69.5
Komiyama et al. [69], 2015	Retrospective analysis	661	79	–
Overall		1,105	76.5–95	51.3–69.5

OS after SBRT in patients with stage I NSCLC judged as operable.
[a] 2a OS.

Expanding the Indication for SBRT

SBRT has been established as the treatment of choice for medically inoperable patients with early-stage NSCLC. Based on the excellent results in this high-risk patient cohort, it is currently strongly debated whether SBRT has a role in fitter and younger patients, who are considered medically operable. Ideally, this question would be addressed and answered in the form of randomized controlled trials. Indeed, 3 randomized trials comparing SBRT and surgical lobectomy have been started, but unfortunately all were stopped very early due to poor accrual. Consequently, no level 1 evidence is available.

However, all existing data point towards a very similar or even equivalent outcome of SBRT and surgery for early-stage NSCLC. Two of the randomized trials mentioned above (STARS, ROSEL) pooled their cohorts, resulting in 58 patients randomized between SBRT and lobectomy [64]. The most relevant difference was the substantially lower toxicity of SBRT: grade 3 toxicity was only observed in 10% after SBRT compared to 44% of the patients suffering from grade 3 or 4 toxicity after lobectomy. No significant differences in the patterns of disease recurrence were observed. Despite the analysis reporting improved OS after SBRT, this interpretation should be taken with caution because of the limitations of the pooled analysis of only a few patients. Very promising and maybe equivalent survival after SBRT compared to surgery is also supported by a growing number of prospective [65] and retrospective studies [46, 66–69], where SBRT was performed in operable patients who refused surgical resection. An overview is given in Table 3.

The results of SBRT in early-stage lung cancer have prompted the question of whether SBRT also has a role in locally advanced stages of disease. The potential role of SBRT is currently evaluated in several ways, where it is integrated into combined radio-chemotherapy: (1) SBRT treatment of the primary tumor while involved nodes are treated with conventionally fractionated radiotherapy [70]; (2) SBRT performed as a boost after conventionally fractionated radiotherapy [71]; (3) SBRT boost only if conventionally fractionated radiotherapy did not achieve complete tumor remission [72], and (4) stereotactic re-irradiation of intrathoracic tumor recurrences after prior radiotherapy in curative intent [73]. So far, only proof of principle trials have been performed and no valid conclusions for clinical practice can be

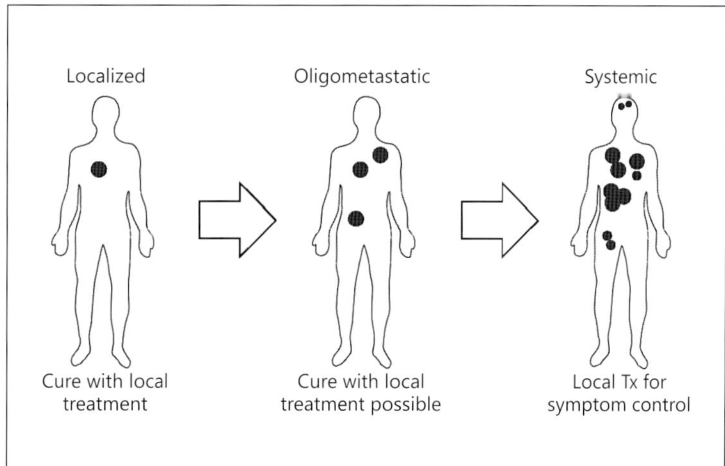

Fig. 4. The concept of oligo-metastases as an intermediate stage between localized disease and diffuse metastatic disease.

drawn. Consequently, the application of SBRT in these situations should be restricted to clinical trials.

SBRT for Oligo-Metastatic Lung Cancer

Definition of Oligo-Metastases
While the term "oligo-metastases" was only introduced in 1995 and revised in 2011 by Hellman and Weichselbaum [74, 75], the concept of local treatment with curative intent in a situation of limited metastatic disease has been practiced for many decades. In this concept, oligo-metastasis is defined as an intermediate stage between localized disease and diffuse metastatic disease (Fig. 4). However, recent preclinical and clinical research have substantially improved our understanding of oligo-metastasis as a distinct stage of disease, which has been evaluated in randomized trials and is recognized in multidisciplinary guidelines. A case example is given is Figure 5.

Most clinical studies defined oligo-metastases purely based on metastatic tumor load: a limited number of metastases (usually a maximum of 3–5) in a limited number of organs (usually a maximum of 1–2). Many studies have confirmed that a lower metastatic tumor volume is associated with improved OS. However, long-term OS is achieved in patients with a higher tumor load as well, indicating that the number of imaging-based metastases independently from the primary cancer and independently from other clinical and biological criteria is not sufficient for precise identification of patients, which will benefit from a local intervention.

Furthermore, the terminology of oligo-metastasis is frequently over- and misused: the identification of "few metastases" represents several very different stages of disease (Fig. 6) with very different prognoses and goals of the local intervention. The immediate goal of local metastasis ablation may be cure in metachronous oligo-metastasis and may be to delay the switch of systemic treatment in oligo-progressive disease. Many early studies did not differentiate between these clinical scenarios, making their interpretation very difficult.

Evidence Supporting the Value of Radiotherapy in Oligo-Metastatic NSCLC
The highest level of evidence is available for oligo-metastatic brain metastases [76]. Patients with 1–3 brain metastases and a good performance status were randomized between whole brain irradiation only (palliative nonradical treatment) and whole

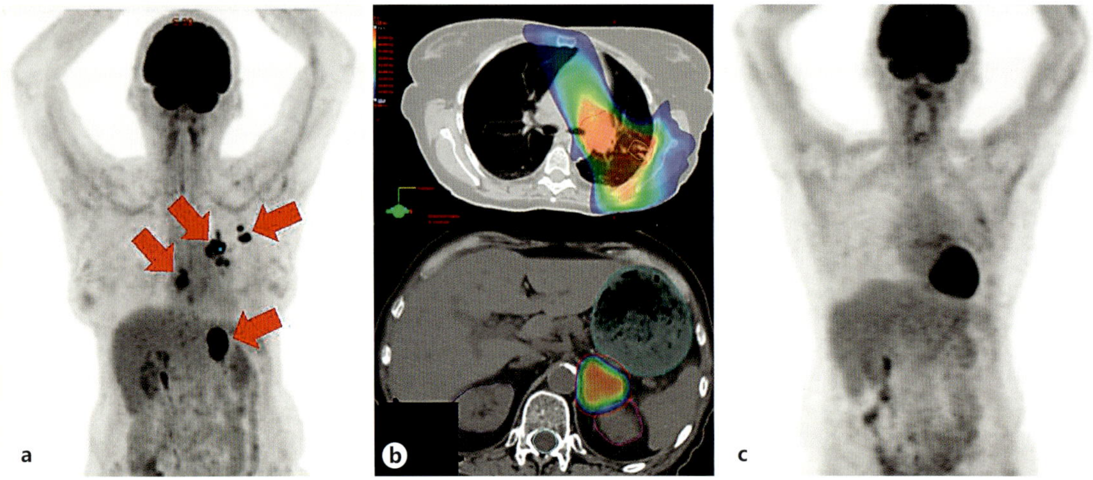

Fig. 5. a Primary diagnosis of oligo-metastatic NSCLC, adenocarcinoma without activating driver mutation. **b** Induction chemotherapy followed by radical radiotherapy. **c** 12-month follow-up with a complete response.

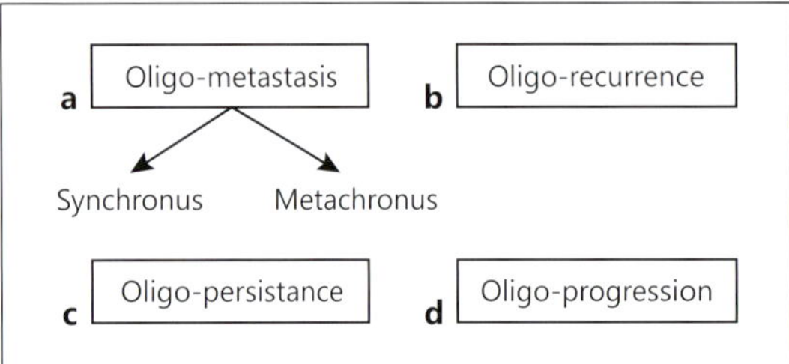

Fig. 6. a Newly developed metastatic disease. **b** Metastatic disease recurrence. **c** Unresponsive subclones/lesions during systemic treatment. **d** Resistance development of subclones/lesions during systemic treatment.

brain irradiation plus radical radiosurgery: of 333 randomized patients, the primary was lung cancer in almost two thirds. Local ablative radiosurgery significantly improved OS by about 2 months in the good-prognosis patients with RPA class 1.

De Ruysscher et al. [77] conducted a prospective phase II trial of radical radiotherapy in patients with synchronous oligo-metastatic NSCLC. About three-quarters of the patients suffered from locoregional stage IIIA and IIIB disease, and >85% of the patients had a solitary metastasis.

The median OS in 39 patients was 13.5 months and median progression-free survival (PFS) was 12.1 months. These results appear similar to stage-matched results in patients without metastatic disease supporting the local radical approach.

Gomez et al. [78] reported a randomized phase II trial in (mostly synchronous) oligo-metastatic NSCLC. The patients were randomized between systemic treatment only and systemic treatment followed by local consolidative therapy. The subjects predominantly had adenocarcinoma, the nodal status was N2/N3 in the majority of the patients, and >60% of the patients had one solitary nonregional metastasis. The study was terminated early after randomization of 49 patients by the Data Safety Monitoring Committee: at a median follow-up time of 12.4 months, the median PFS was 3.9 months versus 11.9 months after systemic treatment only and additional local consolidative treatment, respectively. Most importantly, the local treatment – containing some form of radiotherapy in 96% of all patients – changed the systemic progression pattern: the median time to development of new metastases was prolonged from

5.7 to 11.9 months. Adverse events were similar between groups, with no grade 4 adverse events or deaths due to treatment.

A large meta-analysis of 757 oligo-metastatic NSCLC patients reported a 5a OS rate of 29.4% and the timing of metastatic disease (synchronous vs. metachronous) and intrathoracic nodal status were key determinants of long-term survival [79]. Surgery was the most frequent local treatment modality for the primary tumor (84%) and oligo-metastases (62%). A recent multi-institutional analysis of 907 patients treated with SBRT for pulmonary oligo-metastasis (about a third with NSCLC) reported 5a OS ranging between 24 and 38% [80], which does not appear to be different to results achieved in surgical cohorts [81].

Consequently, current guidelines (ESMO 2016; NCCN v5.2017) recognize the oligo-metastatic state. Whereas the NCCN guideline already recommends a radical local treatment approach, the ESMO guideline is more conservative and recommends treatment within prospective trials. However, the latest data of Gomez et al. [78] were not yet available for both guidelines.

The Optimal Local Intervention to Treat Oligo-Metastatic Disease

Local treatment of oligo-metastases has its longest tradition in colorectal cancer, and resection of liver metastases has achieved long-term survival that is longer than expected in metastatic disease [82]. However, the true value of surgery compared to a treatment strategy without local treatment has never been proven in randomized controlled trials, and many patients are technically unresectable or medically inoperable. Consequently, there is a need for minimally invasive or even noninvasive local treatment methodologies. This is especially important because many patients develop progressive disease after "successful" local treatment of oligo-metastasis, and therefore may require multiple local interventions.

Recently, the CLOCC study reported improved long-term OS after radiofrequency ablation with chemotherapy of unresectable colorectal liver metastases compared to chemotherapy alone [83]. Retrospective comparisons did not observe differences in local tumor control between radiofrequency ablation and surgical resection [84]. Similarly, SBRT today achieves excellent local tumor control targeting metastases at virtually all anatomical locations (lung, liver, bones, lymph nodes, adrenal). The efficacy of SBRT has been shown to be independent from the primary tumor site [28, 85]: metastases of so-called radio-resistant histology can be effectively controlled if sufficiently high radiation doses are applied. Consequently, retrospective comparisons did not observe differences in local metastasis control, disease progression, and OS between surgery and SBRT as local treatment in oligo-metastatic NSCLC [86].

SBRT has several unique strengths, making it highly suitable for the treatment of oligo-metastatic disease: it is delivered noninvasively in 1 or few outpatient treatment sessions; it achieves high rates of local tumor control with low rates of toxicity, and it allows simultaneous treatment of metastases at different anatomical compartments, for example the lungs and liver. Finally, SBRT can be delivered without the need or risk for interruption of systemic treatments [87], which is of particular importance in oncogene-addicted NSCLC under TKI treatment, for example. Even short discontinuation of TKI treatment by a few days bears a very high risk of disease flare [88].

The observations of similar outcomes achieved with different local ablative treatments has led to the development of the so-called toolbox concept for the treatment of colorectal liver metastases in the current ESMO guideline [89]: different local ablative treatment options have distinct pros and cons but may achieve a similar oncological outcome if sufficient expertise is available at the treating institution. Current guidelines (ESMO

2016; NCCN v5.2017) support the use of high-dose radiotherapy and especially SBRT in oligo-metastatic NSCLC. NCCN guidelines recommend treatment of the primary according to the cM0 algorithms and SBRT is described as the "typical" treatment modality together with surgery for the oligo-metastatic sites. Similarly, ESMO guidelines state SBRT and surgery as standard local treatment options in oligo-metastatic NSCLC.

Consequently, SBRT has been the most frequently used local treatment modality in a prospective trial about oligo-metastatic NSCLC: 96% of all patients received some form of radiotherapy and 60% were treated with SBRT, while only 4% were treated with surgery alone [78].

Optimization of Radical Treatment in Oligo-Metastatic NSCLC

Despite aggressive local treatment of all visible tumors – the locoregional primary cancer and all metastases – most patients will develop progressive disease. Gomez et al. [78] and De Ruysscher et al. [77] reported that the progression pattern is distant, with 16/19 and 31/33 of the recurrences located outside the initially involved and locally treated tumor sites.

Several strategies are currently being pursued to improve outcome in oligo-metastatic disease. As the definition of oligo-metastasis is currently based on the number of metastatic lesions, only the accuracy of staging is of utmost importance. A large multi-institutional study reported improved OS in FDG-PET-staged oligo-metastatic lung disease compared to patients without FDG-PET staging [47]. The 2-year OS was 64.8% compared to 52.6%, suggesting that FDG-PET staging should be a mandatory component to select the right patients for radical local treatment.

Several patient and tumor characteristics are well-established prognostic factors after the use of various local treatment modalities for oligo-metastatic disease at various locations. Despite substantial variability between the individual studies, 4 common prognostic categories for improved OS can be extracted: (1) young age; (2) good performance status; (3) slowly progressing cancer, and (4) low overall tumor burden. We have recently reported a nomogram to estimate OS in oligo-metastatic lung disease treated with radical SBRT, achieving differentiation between a poor 2-year OS of 20% and excellent 2-year OS 80% [80]. However, the predictive value of the nomogram remains to be evaluated.

Ideally, patient selection for radical treatment would not only be based on clinical and radiological criteria, but also include biomarkers differentiating between patients with truly oligo-metastatic disease and patients with a systemic disease. However, limited research is currently available in this field and both prospective and independent validation are required [90, 91].

Finally, radical local treatment needs to be integrated into multimodality treatment strategies. Considering the high risk of systemic disease progression after local treatment of oligo-metastases, more effective systemic treatment strategies are urgently needed. First studies are evaluating the combination of SBRT and immunotherapy for oligo-metastatic NSCLC (NCT02086721): SBRT is considered as especially promising because of the synergistic effects of high-dose radiotherapy and immunotherapy [92, 93].

SBRT for Oligo-Progressive Lung Cancer

Definition of Oligo-Progression

Oligo-progression needs to be differentiated from oligo-metastasis. In the oligo-progressive concept, patients may have had widespread systemic disease initially, but after systemic treatment with a partial or complete response, only a limited number of metastases show progression in radiological imaging. Local treatment to all oligo-progressive lesions is thought to eradicate the de-dif-

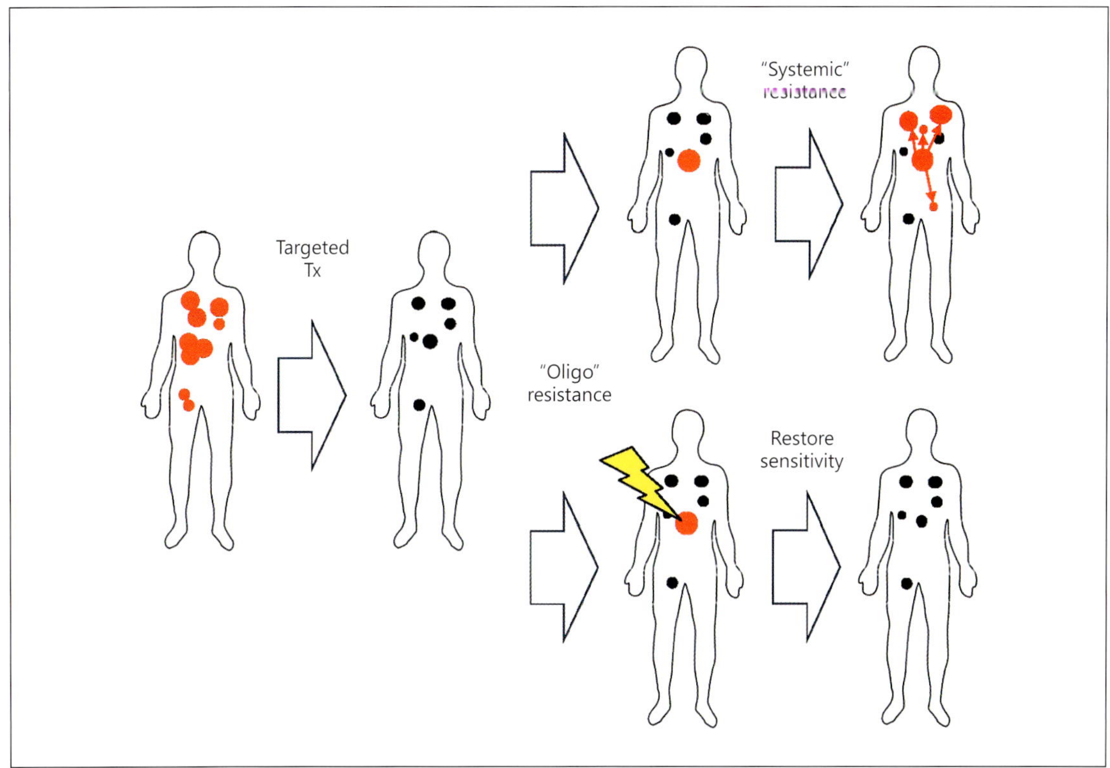

Fig. 7. Rational of local treatment in oligo-progressive disease. Red circles represent progressive metastases, black circles show metastases controlled by (targeted) systemic treatment.

ferentiated clones and restore overall sensitivity of the metastatic disease (Fig. 7).

Local treatment is currently practiced, especially in patients with an activating driver mutation and experiencing oligo-progression during treatment with targeted therapies. Approximately 10–20% of Caucasian and 30–40% of Asian NSCLC adenocarcinoma patients exhibit a somatic mutation in EGFR, with an additional 4–7% of patients having an ALK rearrangement. The frequency is higher in never smokers, women, and patients of East Asian ethnicity [94]. In these molecularly defined populations, targeted therapy using TKIs has produced higher response rates, improved PFS, better tolerability with reduced side effects, and superior quality of life compared with standard platinum-based chemo-

therapy, which has been shown in several randomized trials [95]. Despite initial activity of the TKIs, acquired resistance eventually develops with a median PFS of 8–10 months in patients with ALK rearrangements and 9–13 months in patients with EGFR mutations, and ultimately all patients develop progressive disease [96–100]. This acquired resistance can be attributed to a number of common mechanisms in the majority of cases, although reasons remain unknown in approximately 35% of cases [101–103].

While the concept of oligo-progressive disease implies a potential benefit of local treatment, the question arises of whether this state actually exists in NSCLC [104]. Data from published literature indicates that the proportion of patients progressing with an oligo-progressive pattern of disease ranges from 15 to 47% during EGFR TKI treatment [105–107]. The oligo-progressive disease concept is further supported by data from rebiopsy series, where sites of progression due to TKI resistance are selected in a Darwinian manner and contribute to systemic re-seeding with new sites of distant disease and subsequent widespread disease progression [106, 108, 109].

Outcome of SBRT for Oligo-Progressive Lung Cancer

According to the current ESMO [110] as well as NCCN guidelines, a combined local treatment with continuation of first-line TKI in the setting of oligo-progressive disease is described as a reasonable treatment option with possible improved PFS or even long-term survival. The NCCN guidelines explicitly emphasize the use of definitive radiotherapy, particularly SBRT in these settings if it can be safely delivered.

However, there is currently still limited evidence for the concept of local therapy in oligo-progressive disease, mostly coming from 2 small US single-center retrospective series. In a retrospective study of the Memorial Sloan Kettering group with a total of 184 patients, a series of 18 EGFR-mutated patients with TKI therapy received local therapy for extracranial oligo-progressive disease followed by continuation of TKI. Local therapy was defined as surgery, radiotherapy, or radiofrequency ablation. The median PFS after local therapy was 10 months, the median time to change in systemic therapy was 22 months, and OS was 41 months [105].

The University of Colorado group reported a retrospective series of 65 patients with TKI treatment of either crizotinib or erlotinib who presented with progression in the CNS and/or limited extracranial oligo-progression [106]. A total of 51 of the patients had progressed at the time of analysis, out of which 25 (49%) were deemed suitable for local therapy. The median PFS1 of all patients ($n = 65$) was 10.3 months, while ALK-mutated patients ($n = 38$) had a shorter PFS1 of 9.0 months compared to 13.8 months in EGFR-mutated patients ($n = 27$). Patients with CNS progression ($n = 10$) received local treatment with either SRS (<4 lesions) or WBRT (>4 lesions) and showed a median PFS1 of 10.9 months and PFS2 of 7.1 months. Of these patients, 20% ($n = 2$) did not progress after local treatment, 30% ($n = 3$) progressed in the CNS, and 50% ($n = 5$) showed extracranial progression. Patients with extracranial oligo-progression ($n = 15$) were treated with SBRT in most cases, with a single case of adrenal metastectomy mentioned. PFS1 and PFS2 in these patients were 9.0 and 4.0 months, respectively. Of these patients, 27% ($n = 4$) showed no signs of progression after local treatment, 20% ($n = 3$) progressed in the CNS, and 53% ($n = 8$) showed further extracranial progression.

As a second study with 38 patients, ALK fusion-positive patients developing extracranial oligo-progressive disease ($n = 14$) under treatment with crizotinib were treated with local SBRT or hypofractionated radiotherapy [111]. Local control rates were 100% (6 months) and 86% (12 months) [112].

There was no sign of acute or late grade >2 toxicity. Radiotherapy increased the median overall time on crizotinib to 28 months compared to 10.1 months in patients who did not receive local treatment. OS in patients continuing treatment with crizotinib for >12 months was 72 versus 12% (<12 months; $p = 0.0001$). Median PFS1 for patients receiving local ablative treatment was 14 months compared to 7.2 months in patients who were not eligible to receive local treatment (widespread systemic disease, poor Karnofsky Performance Status, or oligo-progressive disease) and switched to alternative systemic therapy. The median PFS2 was 5.5 months and was longer in patients with 1–2 lesions (7 months) compared to 3–4 lesions (2 months; $p = 0.12$).

However, the absence of randomization limits interpretation of these studies. A randomized study with an appropriate control group is therefore required in order to effectively evaluate the true benefit of adding SBRT to TKI therapy in patients with oligo progressive disease [110, 113, 114].

Conclusion

Stereotactic radiotherapy has become an essential component of lung cancer care. The unique characteristics of SBRT – its noninvasive nature, practice as an outpatient procedure in few sessions, the highly favorable therapeutic ratio with low toxicity and excellent local tumor control – have established SBRT as a guideline-recommended treatment in several situations and indications for lung cancer. Simultaneously, limitations and challenges of SBRT have been identified. A deep understanding of the experiences made in the field of lung cancer are essential when SBRT is transferred to other cancer sites.

References

1 Lax I, Blomgren H, Naslund I, Svanstrom R: Stereotactic radiotherapy of malignancies in the abdomen. Methodological aspects. Acta Oncol 1994;33: 677–683.
2 Uematsu M, Shioda A, Tahara K, Fukui T, Yamamoto F, Tsumatori G, Ozeki Y, Aoki T, Watanabe M, Kusano S: Focal, high dose, and fractionated modified stereotactic radiation therapy for lung carcinoma patients: a preliminary experience. Cancer 1998;82:1062–1070.
3 Wulf J, Hadinger U, Oppitz U, Olshausen B, Flentje M: Stereotactic radiotherapy of extracranial targets: CT-simulation and accuracy of treatment in the stereotactic body frame. Radiother Oncol 2000;57:225–236.
4 Herfarth KK, Debus J, Lohr F, Bahner ML, Fritz P, Hoss A, Schlegel W, Wannenmacher MF. Extracranial stereotactic radiation therapy: set-up accuracy of patients treated for liver metastases. Int J Radiat Oncol Biol Phys 2000;46:329–335.
5 Pan H, Simpson DR, Mell LK, Mundt AJ, Lawson JD: A survey of stereotactic body radiotherapy use in the United States. Cancer 2011;117:4566–4572.
6 Ramella S, Maranzano E, Frata P, Mantovani C, Lazzari G, Menichelli C, Navarria P, Pergolizzi S, Salvi F: Radiotherapy in Italy for non-small cell lung cancer: patterns of care survey. Tumori 2012;98:66–78.
7 Benedict SH, Yenice KM, Followill D, Galvin JM, Hinson W, Kavanagh B, Keall P, Lovelock M, Meeks S, Papiez L, et al: Stereotactic body radiation therapy: the report of AAPM Task Group 101. Med Phys 2010;37:4078–4101.
8 Potters L, Kavanagh B, Galvin JM, Hevezi JM, Janjan NA, Larson DA, Mehta MP, Ryu S, Steinberg M, Timmerman R, et al: American Society for Therapeutic Radiology and Oncology (ASTRO) and American College of Radiology (ACR) practice guideline for the performance of stereotactic body radiation therapy. Int J Radiat Oncol Biol Phys 2010;76:326–332.
9 Sahgal A, Roberge D, Schellenberg D, Purdie TG, Swaminath A, Pantarotto J, Filion E, Gabos Z, Butler J, Letourneau D, et al: The Canadian Association of Radiation Oncology scope of practice guidelines for lung, liver and spine stereotactic body radiotherapy. Clin Oncol 2012;24:629–639.
10 Kirkbride P, Cooper T: Stereotactic body radiotherapy: guidelines for commissioners, providers and clinicians: a national report. Clin Oncol 2011;23:163–164.
11 Guckenberger M, Andratschke N, Alheit H, Holy R, Moustakis C, Nestle U, Sauer O, Deutschen Gesellschaft fur Radioonkologie (DEGRO): Definition of stereotactic body radiotherapy: principles and practice for the treatment of stage I non-small cell lung cancer. Strahlenther Onkol 2014;190:26–33.
12 Loo BW, Chang JY, Dawson LA, Kavanagh BD, Koong AC, Senan S, Timmerman RD: Stereotactic ablative radiotherapy: what's in a name? Pract Radiat Oncol 2011;1:38–39.
13 McGarry RC, Papiez L, Williams M, Whitford T, Timmerman RD: Stereotactic body radiation therapy of early-stage non-small-cell lung carcinoma: phase I study. Int J Radiat Oncol Biol Phys 2005; 63:1010–1015.
14 Senthi S, Haasbeek CJ, Slotman BJ, Senan S: Outcomes of stereotactic ablative radiotherapy for central lung tumours: a systematic review. Radiother Oncol 2013;106:276–282.
15 Goldstraw P, Chansky K, Crowley J, Rami-Porta R, Asamura H, Eberhardt WE, Nicholson AG, Groome P, Mitchell A, Bolejack V, et al: The IASLC Lung Cancer Staging Project: proposals for revision of the TNM stage groupings in the forthcoming (eighth) edition of the TNM Classification for Lung Cancer. J Thorac Oncol 2016;11:39–51.
16 Raz DJ, Zell JA, Ou SH, Gandara DR, Anton-Culver H, Jablons DM: Natural history of stage I non-small cell lung cancer: implications for early detection. Chest 2007;132:193–199.
17 Kravchenko J, Berry M, Arbeev K, Lyerly HK, Yashin A, Akushevich I: Cardiovascular comorbidities and survival of lung cancer patients: Medicare data based analysis. Lung Cancer 2015;88: 85–93.

18 Eguchi T, Bains S, Lee MC, Tan KS, Hristov B, Buitrago DH, Bains MS, Downey RJ, Huang J, Isbell JM, et al: Impact of increasing age on cause-specific mortality and morbidity in patients with stage I non-small-cell lung cancer: a competing risks analysis. J Clin Oncol 2017;35:281–290.

19 Rowell NP, Williams CJ: Radical radiotherapy for stage I/II non-small cell lung cancer in patients not sufficiently fit for or declining surgery (medically inoperable). Cochrane Database Syst Rev 2001; 2:CD002935.

20 Nagata Y, Takayama K, Matsuo Y, Norihisa Y, Mizowaki T, Sakamoto T, Sakamoto M, Mitsumori M, Shibuya K, Araki N, et al: Clinical outcomes of a phase I/II study of 48 Gy of stereotactic body radiotherapy in 4 fractions for primary lung cancer using a stereotactic body frame. Int J Radiat Oncol Biol Phys 2005;63:1427–1431.

21 Fakiris AJ, McGarry RC, Yiannoutsos CT, Papiez L, Williams M, Henderson MA, Timmerman R: Stereotactic body radiation therapy for early-stage non-small-cell lung carcinoma: four-year results of a prospective phase II study. Int J Radiat Oncol Biol Phys 2009;75: 677–682.

22 Ricardi U, Filippi AR, Guarneri A, Giglioli FR, Ciammella P, Franco P, Mantovani C, Borasio P, Scagliotti GV, Ragona R: Stereotactic body radiation therapy for early stage non-small cell lung cancer: results of a prospective trial. Lung Cancer 2010;68:72–77.

23 Timmerman R, Paulus R, Galvin J, Michalski J, Straube W, Bradley J, Fakiris A, Bezjak A, Videtic G, Johnstone D, et al: Stereotactic body radiation therapy for inoperable early stage lung cancer. JAMA 2010;303:1070–1076.

24 Bral S, Gevaert T, Linthout N, Versmessen H, Collen C, Engels B, Verdries D, Everaert H, Christian N, De Ridder M, et al: Prospective, risk-adapted strategy of stereotactic body radiotherapy for early-stage non-small-cell lung cancer: results of a Phase II trial. Int J Radiat Oncol Biol Phys 2011;80:1343–1349.

25 Lindberg K, Nyman J, Riesenfeld Kallskog V, Hoyer M, Lund JA, Lax I, Wersall P, Karlsson K, Friesland S, Lewensohn R: Long-term results of a prospective phase II trial of medically inoperable stage I NSCLC treated with SBRT – the Nordic experience. Acta Oncol 2015;54:1–9.

26 Sun B, Brooks ED, Komaki RU, Liao Z, Jeter MD, McAleer MF, Allen PK, Balter PA, Welsh JD, O'Reilly MS, et al: 7-year follow-up after stereotactic ablative radiotherapy for patients with stage I non-small cell lung cancer: results of a phase 2 clinical trial. Cancer 2017;123:3031–3039.

27 Guckenberger M, Wulf J, Mueller G, Krieger T, Baier K, Gabor M, Richter A, Wilbert J, Flentje M: Dose-response relationship for image-guided stereotactic body radiotherapy of pulmonary tumors: relevance of 4D dose calculation. Int J Radiat Oncol Biol Phys 2009;74: 47–54.

28 Guckenberger M, Klement RJ, Allgauer M, Andratschke N, Blanck O, Boda-Heggemann J, Dieckmann K, Duma M, Ernst I, Ganswindt U, et al: Local tumor control probability modeling of primary and secondary lung tumors in stereotactic body radiotherapy. Radiother Oncol 2016;118:485–491.

29 Kestin L, Grills I, Guckenberger M, Belderbos J, Hope AJ, Werner-Wasik M, Sonke JJ, Bissonnette JP, Xiao Y, Yan D, et al: Dose-response relationship with clinical outcome for lung stereotactic body radiotherapy (SBRT) delivered via online image guidance. Radiother Oncol 2014;110:499–504.

30 Guckenberger M, Allgauer M, Appold S, Dieckmann K, Ernst I, Ganswindt U, Holy R, Nestle U, Nevinny-Stickel M, Semrau S, et al: Safety and efficacy of stereotactic body radiotherapy for stage I non-small-cell lung cancer in routine clinical practice: a patterns-of-care and outcome analysis. J Thorac Oncol 2013; 8:1050–1058.

31 Kirkpatrick JP, Brenner DJ, Orton CG: Point/counterpoint: the linear-quadratic model is inappropriate to model high dose per fraction effects in radiosurgery. Med Phys 2009;36:3381–3384.

32 Guckenberger M, Klement RJ, Allgauer M, Appold S, Dieckmann K, Ernst I, Ganswindt U, Holy R, Nestle U, Nevinny-Stickel M, et al: Applicability of the linear-quadratic formalism for modeling local tumor control probability in high dose per fraction stereotactic body radiotherapy for early stage non-small cell lung cancer. Radiother Oncol 2013;109: 13–20.

33 Shuryak I, Carlson DJ, Brown JM, Brenner DJ: High-dose and fractionation effects in stereotactic radiation therapy: analysis of tumor control data from 2,965 patients. Radiother Oncol 2015;115:327–334.

34 Kopek N, Paludan M, Petersen J, Hansen AT, Grau C, Hoyer M: Co-morbidity index predicts for mortality after stereotactic body radiotherapy for medically inoperable early-stage non-small cell lung cancer. Radiother Oncol 2009;93: 402–407.

35 Dong M, Liu J, Sun X, Xing L: Prognositc significance of SUV_{max} on pretreatment ^{18}F-FDG PET/CT in early-stage non-small cell lung cancer treated with stereotactic body radiotherapy: a meta-analysis. J Med Imaging Radiat Oncol 2017;61:652–659.

36 Yamamoto T, Kadoya N, Shirata Y, Koto M, Sato K, Matsushita H, Sugawara T, Umezawa R, Kubozono M, Ishikawa Y, et al: Impact of tumor attachment to the pleura measured by a pretreatment CT image on outcome of stage I NSCLC treated with stereotactic body radiotherapy. Radiat Oncol 2015;10:35.

37 Shultz DB, Trakul N, Abelson JA, Murphy JD, Maxim PG, Le QT, Loo BW Jr, Diehn M: Imaging features associated with disease progression after stereotactic ablative radiotherapy for stage I non-small-cell lung cancer. Clin Lung Cancer 2014;15:294–301.e3.

38 Timmerman R, McGarry R, Yiannoutsos C, Papiez L, Tudor K, DeLuca J, Ewing M, Abdulrahman R, DesRosiers C, Williams M, et al: Excessive toxicity when treating central tumors in a phase II study of stereotactic body radiation therapy for medically inoperable early-stage lung cancer. J Clin Oncol 2006;24: 4833–4839.

39 Guckenberger M, Baier K, Polat B, Richter A, Krieger T, Wilbert J, Mueller G, Flentje M: Dose-response relationship for radiation-induced pneumonitis after pulmonary stereotactic body radiotherapy. Radiother Oncol 2010;97:65–70.

40 Ferrero C, Badellino S, Filippi AR, Focaraccio L, Giaj Levra M, Levis M, Moretto F, Torchio R, Ricardi U, Novello S: Pulmonary function and quality of life after VMAT-based stereotactic ablative radiotherapy for early stage inoperable NSCLC: a prospective study. Lung Cancer 2015;89:350–356.

41 van der Voort van Zyp NC, Prevost JB, van der Holt B, Braat C, van Klaveren RJ, Pattynama PM, Levendag PC, Nuyttens JJ: Quality of life after stereotactic radiotherapy for stage I non-small-cell lung cancer. Int J Radiat Oncol Biol Phys 2010;77:31–37.

42 Lagerwaard FJ, Aaronson NK, Gundy CM, Haasbeek CJ, Slotman BJ, Senan S: Patient-reported quality of life after stereotactic ablative radiotherapy for early-stage lung cancer. J Thorac Oncol 2012;7:1148–1154.

43 Guckenberger M, Kestin LL, Hope AJ, Belderbos J, Werner-Wasik M, Yan D, Sonke JJ, Bissonnette JP, Wilbert J, Xiao Y, et al: Is there a lower limit of pretreatment pulmonary function for safe and effective stereotactic body radiotherapy for early-stage non-small cell lung cancer? J Thorac Oncol 2012;7:542–551.

44 Senthi S, Lagerwaard FJ, Haasbeek CJ, Slotman BJ, Senan S: Patterns of disease recurrence after stereotactic ablative radiotherapy for early stage non-small-cell lung cancer: a retrospective analysis. Lancet Oncol 2012;13:802–809.

45 Zhao L, Zhou S, Balter P, Shen C, Gomez DR, Welsh JD, Lin SH, Chang JY: Planning target volume D95 and mean dose should be considered for optimal local control for stereotactic ablative radiation therapy. Int J Radiat Oncol Biol Phys 2016;95:1226–1235.

46 Grills IS, Hope AJ, Guckenberger M, Kestin LL, Werner-Wasik M, Yan D, Sonke JJ, Bissonnette JP, Wilbert J, Xiao Y, et al: A collaborative analysis of stereotactic lung radiotherapy outcomes for early-stage non-small-cell lung cancer using daily online cone-beam computed tomography image-guided radiotherapy. J Thorac Oncol 2012;7:1382–1393.

47 Rieber J, Abbassi-Senger N, Adebahr S, Andratschke N, Blanck O, Duma M, Eble MJ, Ernst I, Flentje M, Gerum S, et al: Influence of institutional experience and technological advances on outcome of stereotactic body radiation therapy for oligometastatic lung disease. Int J Radiat Oncol Biol Phys 2017;98:511–520.

48 Koshy M, Malik R, Mahmood U, Husain Z, Sher DJ: Stereotactic body radiotherapy and treatment at a high volume facility is associated with improved survival in patients with inoperable stage I non-small cell lung cancer. Radiother Oncol 2015;114:148–154.

49 Verstegen NE, Lagerwaard FJ, Haasbeek CJ, Slotman BJ, Senan S: Outcomes of stereotactic ablative radiotherapy following a clinical diagnosis of stage I NSCLC: comparison with a contemporaneous cohort with pathologically proven disease. Radiother Oncol 2011;101:250–254.

50 Stiles BM, Servais EL, Lee PC, Port JL, Paul S, Altorki NK: Point: Clinical stage IA non-small cell lung cancer determined by computed tomography and positron emission tomography is frequently not pathologic IA non-small cell lung cancer: the problem of understaging. J Thorac Cardiovasc Surg 2009;137:13–19.

51 Park HK, Jeon K, Koh WJ, Suh GY, Kim H, Kwon OJ, Chung MP, Lee KS, Shim YM, Han J, et al: Occult nodal metastasis in patients with non-small cell lung cancer at clinical stage IA by PET/CT. Respirology 2010;15:1179–1184.

52 Guckenberger M, Heilman K, Wulf J, Mueller G, Beckmann G, Flentje M: Pulmonary injury and tumor response after stereotactic body radiotherapy (SBRT): results of a serial follow-up CT study. Radiother Oncol 2007;85:435–442.

53 Peulen H, Mantel F, Guckenberger M, Belderbos J, Werner-Wasik M, Hope A, Giuliani M, Grills I, Sonke JJ: Validation of high-risk computed tomography features for detection of local recurrence after stereotactic body radiation therapy for early-stage non-small cell lung cancer. Int J Radiat Oncol Biol Phys 2016;96:134–141.

54 Palma D, Lagerwaard F, Rodrigues G, Haasbeek C, Senan S: Curative treatment of stage I non-small-cell lung cancer in patients with severe COPD: stereotactic radiotherapy outcomes and systematic review. Int J Radiat Oncol Biol Phys 2012;82:1149–1156.

55 Bahig H, Filion E, Vu T, Chalaoui J, Lambert L, Roberge D, Gagnon M, Fortin B, Beliveau-Nadeau D, Mathieu D, et al: Severe radiation pneumonitis after lung stereotactic ablative radiation therapy in patients with interstitial lung disease. Pract Radiat Oncol 2016;6:367–374.

56 Yoshitake T, Shioyama Y, Asai K, Nakamura K, Sasaki T, Ohga S, Kamitani T, Yamaguchi T, Ohshima K, Matsumoto K, et al: Impact of interstitial changes on radiation pneumonitis after stereotactic body radiation therapy for lung cancer. Anticancer Res 2015;35:4909–4913.

57 Ueki N, Matsuo Y, Togashi Y, Kubo T, Shibuya K, Iizuka Y, Mizowaki T, Togashi K, Mishima M, Hiraoka M: Impact of pretreatment interstitial lung disease on radiation pneumonitis and survival after stereotactic body radiation therapy for lung cancer. J Thorac Oncol 2015;10:116–125.

58 Schanne DH, Nestle U, Allgauer M, Andratschke N, Appold S, Dieckmann U, Ernst I, Ganswindt U, Grosu AL, Holy R, et al: Stereotactic body radiotherapy for centrally located stage I NSCLC: a multicenter analysis. Strahlenther Onkol 2015;191:125–132.

59 Verma V, Shostrom VK, Kumar SS, Zhen W, Hallemeier CL, Braunstein SE, Holland J, Harkenrider MM, A SI, Neboori HJ, et al: Multi-institutional experience of stereotactic body radiotherapy for large (≥5 centimeters) non-small cell lung tumors. Cancer 2017;123:688–696.

60 Verma V, Shostrom VK, Zhen W, Zhang M, Braunstein SE, Holland J, Hallemeier CL, Harkenrider MM, Iskhanian A, Jabbour SK, et al: Influence of fractionation scheme and tumor location on toxicities after stereotactic body radiation therapy for large (≥5 cm) non-small cell lung cancer: a multi-institutional analysis. Int J Radiat Oncol Biol Phys 2017;97:778–785.

61 Tekatli H, van 't Hof S, Nossent EJ, Dahele M, Verbakel WF, Slotman BJ, Senan S: Use of stereotactic ablative radiotherapy (SABR) in non-small cell lung cancer measuring more than 5 cm. J Thorac Oncol 2017;12:974–982.

62 Owen D, Olivier KR, Mayo CS, Miller RC, Nelson K, Bauer H, Brown PD, Park SS, Ma DJ, Garces YI: Outcomes of stereotactic body radiotherapy (SBRT) treatment of multiple synchronous and recurrent lung nodules. Radiat Oncol 2015;10:43.

63 Creach KM, Bradley JD, Mahasittiwat P, Robinson CG: Stereotactic body radiation therapy in the treatment of multiple primary lung cancers. Radiother Oncol 2012;104:19–22.

64 Chang JY, Senan S, Paul MA, Mehran RJ, Louie AV, Balter P, Groen HJ, McRae SE, Widder J, Feng L, et al: Stereotactic ablative radiotherapy versus lobectomy for operable stage I non-small-cell lung cancer: a pooled analysis of two randomised trials. Lancet Oncol 2015;16: 630–637.

65 Nagata Y, Hiraoka M, Shibata T, Onishi H, Kokubo M, Karasawa K, Shioyama Y, Onimaru R, Kozuka T, Kunieda E, et al: Prospective trial of stereotactic body radiation therapy for both operable and inoperable T1N0M0 non-small cell lung cancer: Japan Clinical Oncology Group Study JCOG0403. Int J Radiat Oncol Biol Phys 2015;93:989–996.

66 Uematsu M, Shioda A, Suda A, Fukui T, Ozeki Y, Hama Y, Wong JR, Kusano S: Computed tomography-guided frameless stereotactic radiotherapy for stage I non-small cell lung cancer: a 5-year experience. Int J Radiat Oncol Biol Phys 2001;51:666–670.

67 Lagerwaard FJ, Verstegen NE, Haasbeek CJ, Slotman BJ, Paul MA, Smit EF, Senan S: Outcomes of stereotactic ablative radiotherapy in patients with potentially operable stage I non-small cell lung cancer. Int J Radiat Oncol Biol Phys 2012;83:348–353.

68 Onishi H, Shirato H, Nagata Y, Hiraoka M, Fujino M, Gomi K, Karasawa K, Hayakawa K, Niibe Y, Takai Y, et al: Stereotactic body radiotherapy (SBRT) for operable stage I non-small-cell lung cancer: can SBRT be comparable to surgery? Int J Radiat Oncol Biol Phys 2011; 81:1352–1358.

69 Komiyama T, Onishi H, Shioyama Y, Matsumoto Y, Takayama K, Matsuo Y, Miyakawa A, Yamashita H, Nihei K, Matsushita H, et al: Japanese multicenter study of stereotactic body radiotherapy for 661 medically operable patients with stage I non-small cell lung cancer. J Thorac Oncol 2015;10:S210–S211.

70 Chi A, Wen S, Monga M, Almubarak M, He X, Rojanasakul Y, Tse W, Remick SC: Definitive upfront stereotactic ablative radiotherapy combined with image-guided, intensity modulated radiotherapy (IG-IMRT) or IG-IMRT alone for locally advanced non-small cell lung cancer. PLoS One 2016;11:e0162453.

71 Hepel JT, Leonard KL, Safran H, Ng T, Taber A, Khurshid H, Birnbaum A, Wazer DE, DiPetrillo T; Brown University Oncology Research Group: Stereotactic body radiation therapy boost after concurrent chemoradiation for locally advanced non-small cell lung cancer: a phase 1 dose escalation study. Int J Radiat Oncol Biol Phys 2016;96:1021–1027.

72 Feddock J, Arnold SM, Shelton BJ, Sinha P, Conrad G, Chen L, Rinehart J, McGarry RC: Stereotactic body radiation therapy can be used safely to boost residual disease in locally advanced non-small cell lung cancer: a prospective study. Int J Radiat Oncol Biol Phys 2013;85:1325–1331.

73 De Bari B, Filippi AR, Mazzola R, Bonomo P, Trovo M, Livi L, Alongi F: Available evidence on re-irradiation with stereotactic ablative radiotherapy following high-dose previous thoracic radiotherapy for lung malignancies. Cancer Treat Rev 2015;41:511–518.

74 Hellman S, Weichselbaum RR: Oligometastases. J Clin Oncol 1995;13:8–10.

75 Weichselbaum RR, Hellman S: Oligometastases revisited. Nat Rev Clin Oncol 2011;8:378–382.

76 Andrews DW, Scott CB, Sperduto PW, Flanders AE, Gaspar LE, Schell MC, Werner-Wasik M, Demas W, Ryu J, Bahary JP, et al: Whole brain radiation therapy with or without stereotactic radiosurgery boost for patients with one to three brain metastases: phase III results of the RTOG 9508 randomised trial. Lancet 2004;363:1665–1672.

77 De Ruysscher D, Wanders R, van Baardwijk A, Dingemans AM, Reymen B, Houben R, Bootsma G, Pitz C, van Eijsden L, Geraedts W, et al: Radical treatment of non-small-cell lung cancer patients with synchronous oligometastases: long-term results of a prospective phase II trial (Nct01282450). J Thorac Oncol 2012;7:1547–1555.

78 Gomez DR, Blumenschein GR, Jr., Lee JJ, Hernandez M, Ye R, Camidge DR, Doebele RC, Skoulidis F, Gaspar LE, Gibbons DL, et al: Local consolidative therapy versus maintenance therapy or observation for patients with oligometastatic non-small-cell lung cancer without progression after first-line systemic therapy: a multicentre, randomised, controlled, phase 2 study. Lancet Oncol 2016;17:1672–1682.

79 Ashworth AB, Senan S, Palma DA, Riquet M, Chan Ahn Y, Ricardi U, Congedo MT, Gomez DR, Wright GM, Melloni G, et al: An individual patient data metaanalysis of outcomes and prognostic factors after treatment of oligometastatic non-small-cell lung cancer. Clin Lung Cancer 2014;15:346–355.

80 Tanadini-Lang S, Rieber J, Filippi AR, Fode MM, Streblow J, Adebahr S, Andratschke N, Blanck O, Boda-Heggemann J, Duma M, et al: Nomogram based overall survival prediction in stereotactic body radiotherapy for oligo-metastatic lung disease. Radiother Oncol 2017;123:182–188.

81 Pastorino U, Buyse M, Friedel G, Ginsberg RJ, Girard P, Goldstraw P, Johnston M, McCormack P, Pass H, Putnam JB, Jr., et al: Long-term results of lung metastasectomy: prognostic analyses based on 5,206 cases. J Thorac Cardiovasc Surg 1997;113:37–49.

82 Fong Y, Fortner J, Sun RL, Brennan MF, Blumgart LH: Clinical score for predicting recurrence after hepatic resection for metastatic colorectal cancer: analysis of 1,001 consecutive cases. Ann Surg 1999;230:309–321.

83 Ruers T, Punt CJA, van Coevorden F, Pierie JP, Rinkes IB, Ledermann JA, Poston GJ, Bechstein WO, Lentz MA, Mauer ME, et al: Radiofrequency ablation (RFA) combined with chemotherapy for unresectable colorectal liver metastases (CRC LM): long-term survival results of a randomized phase II study of the EORTC-NCRI CCSG-ALM Intergroup 40004 (CLOCC). J Clin Oncol 2015;33.

84 Tanis E, Nordlinger B, Mauer M, Sorbye H, van Coevorden F, Gruenberger T, Schlag PM, Punt CJ, Ledermann J, Ruers TJ: Local recurrence rates after radiofrequency ablation or resection of colorectal liver metastases. Analysis of the European Organisation for Research and Treatment of Cancer #40004 and #40983. Eur J Cancer 2014;50:912–919.

85 Klement RJ, Guckenberger M, Alheid H, Allgauer M, Becker G, Blanck O, Boda-Heggemann J, Brunner T, Duma M, Gerum S, et al: Stereotactic body radiotherapy for oligo-metastatic liver disease – influence of pre-treatment chemotherapy and histology on local tumor control. Radiother Oncol 2017;123:227–233.

86 Widder J, Klinkenberg TJ, Ubbels JF, Wiegman EM, Groen HJ, Langendijk JA: Pulmonary oligometastases: metastasectomy or stereotactic ablative radiotherapy? Radiother Oncol 2013;107:409–413.

87 Kroeze SG, Fritz C, Hoyer M, Lo SS, Ricardi U, Sahgal A, Stahel R, Stupp R, Guckenberger M: Toxicity of concurrent stereotactic radiotherapy and targeted therapy or immunotherapy: a systematic review. Cancer Treat Rev 2017;53:25–37.

88 Chaft JE, Oxnard GR, Sima CS, Kris MG, Miller VA, Riely GJ: Disease flare after tyrosine kinase inhibitor discontinuation in patients with EGFR-mutant lung cancer and acquired resistance to erlotinib or gefitinib: implications for clinical trial design. Clin Cancer Res 2011;17:6298–6303.

89 van Cutsem E, Cervantes A, Adam R, Sobrero A, Van Krieken JH, Aderka D, Aranda Aguilar E, Bardelli A, Benson A, Bodoky G, et al: ESMO consensus guidelines for the management of patients with metastatic colorectal cancer. Ann Oncol 2016;27:1386–1422.

90 Lussier YA, Xing HR, Salama JK, Khodarev NN, Huang Y, Zhang Q, Khan SA, Yang X, Hasselle MD, Darga TE, et al: MicroRNA expression characterizes oligometastasis(es). PLoS One 2011;6:e28650.

91 Wong AC, Watson SP, Pitroda SP, Son CH, Das LC, Stack ME, Uppal A, Oshima G, Khodarev NN, Salama JK, et al: Clinical and molecular markers of long-term survival after oligometastasis-directed stereotactic body radiotherapy (SBRT). Cancer 2016;122:2242–2250.

92 Twyman-Saint Victor C, Rech AJ, Maity A, Rengan R, Pauken KE, Stelekati E, Benci JL, Xu B, Dada H, Odorizzi PM, et al: Radiation and dual checkpoint blockade activate non-redundant immune mechanisms in cancer. Nature 2015;520:373–377.

93 Bernstein MB, Krishnan S, Hodge JW, Chang JY: Immunotherapy and stereotactic ablative radiotherapy (ISABR): a curative approach? Nat Rev Clin Oncol 2016;13:516–524.

94 Lovly C, Horn L, Pao W: Molecular profiling of lung cancer. My Cancer Genome. Updated March 28, 2016. www.mycancergenome.org/content/disease/lung-cancer/.

95 Lee JK, Hahn S, Kim DW, Suh KJ, Keam B, Kim TM, Lee SH, Heo DS: Epidermal growth factor receptor tyrosine kinase inhibitors vs conventional chemotherapy in non-small cell lung cancer harboring wild-type epidermal growth factor receptor: a meta-analysis. JAMA 2014;311:1430–1437.

96 Mok TS, Wu YL, Thongprasert S, Yang CH, Chu DT, Saijo N, Sunpaweravong P, Han B, Margono B, Ichinose Y, et al: Gefitinib or carboplatin-paclitaxel in pulmonary adenocarcinoma. N Engl J Med 2009;361:947–957.

97 Rosell R, Carcereny E, Gervais R, Vergnenegre A, Massuti B, Felip E, Palmero R, Garcia-Gomez R, Pallares C, Sanchez JM, et al: Erlotinib versus standard chemotherapy as first-line treatment for European patients with advanced EGFR mutation-positive non-small-cell lung cancer (EURTAC): a multicentre, open-label, randomised phase 3 trial. Lancet Oncol 2012;13:239–246.

98 Sequist LV, Yang JC, Yamamoto N, O'Byrne K, Hirsh V, Mok T, Geater SL, Orlov S, Tsai CM, Boyer M, et al: Phase III study of afatinib or cisplatin plus pemetrexed in patients with metastatic lung adenocarcinoma with EGFR mutations. J Clin Oncol 2013;31:3327–3334.

99 Shaw AT, Kim DW, Nakagawa K, Seto T, Crino L, Ahn MJ, De Pas T, Besse B, Solomon BJ, Blackhall F, et al: Crizotinib versus chemotherapy in advanced ALK-positive lung cancer. N Engl J Med 2013;368:2385–2394.

100 Solomon BJ, Mok T, Kim DW, Wu YL, Nakagawa K, Mekhail T, Felip E, Cappuzzo F, Paolini J, Usari T, et al: First-line crizotinib versus chemotherapy in ALK-positive lung cancer. N Engl J Med 2014;371:2167–2177.

101 Engelman JA, Janne PA: Mechanisms of acquired resistance to epidermal growth factor receptor tyrosine kinase inhibitors in non-small cell lung cancer. Clin Cancer Res 2008;14:2895–2899.

102 Gainor JF, Shaw AT: Emerging paradigms in the development of resistance to tyrosine kinase inhibitors in lung cancer. J Clin Oncol 2013;31:3987–3996.

103 Sequist LV, Waltman BA, Dias-Santagata D, Digumarthy S, Turke AB, Fidias P, Bergethon K, Shaw AT, Gettinger S, Cosper AK, et al: Genotypic and histological evolution of lung cancers acquiring resistance to EGFR inhibitors. Sci Transl Med 2011;3:75ra26.

104 Ashworth A, Rodrigues G, Boldt G, Palma D: Is there an oligometastatic state in non-small cell lung cancer? A systematic review of the literature. Lung Cancer 2013;82:197–203.

105 Yu HA, Sima CS, Huang J, Solomon SB, Rimner A, Paik P, Pietanza MC, Azzoli CG, Rizvi NA, Krug LM, et al: Local therapy with continued EGFR tyrosine kinase inhibitor therapy as a treatment strategy in EGFR-mutant advanced lung cancers that have developed acquired resistance to EGFR tyrosine kinase inhibitors. J Thorac Oncol 2013;8:346–351.

106 Weickhardt AJ, Scheier B, Burke JM, Gan G, Lu X, Bunn PA, Jr., Aisner DL, Gaspar LE, Kavanagh BD, Doebele RC, et al: Local ablative therapy of oligoprogressive disease prolongs disease control by tyrosine kinase inhibitors in oncogene-addicted non-small-cell lung cancer. J Thorac Oncol 2012;7:1807–1814.

107 Yoshida T, Yoh K, Niho S, Umemura S, Matsumoto S, Ohmatsu H, Ohe Y, Goto K: RECIST progression patterns during EGFR tyrosine kinase inhibitor treatment of advanced non-small cell lung cancer patients harboring an EGFR mutation. Lung Cancer 2015;90:477–483.

108 Kuiper JL, Heideman DA, Thunnissen E, Paul MA, van Wijk AW, Postmus PE, Smit EF: Incidence of T790M mutation in (sequential) rebiopsies in EGFR-mutated NSCLC-patients. Lung Cancer 2014;85:19–24.

109 Al-Halabi H, Sayegh K, Digamurthy SR, Niemierko A, Piotrowska Z, Willers H, Sequist LV: Pattern of failure analysis in metastatic EGFR-mutant lung cancer treated with tyrosine kinase inhibitors to identify candidates for consolidation stereotactic body radiation therapy. J Thorac Oncol 2015;10:1601–1607.

110 Novello S, Barlesi F, Califano R, Cufer T, Ekman S, Levra MG, Kerr K, Popat S, Reck M, Senan S, et al: Metastatic non-small-cell lung cancer: ESMO clinical practice guidelines for diagnosis, treatment and follow-up. Ann Oncol 2016;27(suppl 5):v1–v27.

111 Gan GN, Weickhardt AJ, Scheier B, Doebele RC, Gaspar LE, Kavanagh BD, Camidge DR: Stereotactic radiation therapy can safely and durably control sites of extra-central nervous system oligoprogressive disease in anaplastic lymphoma kinase-positive lung cancer patients receiving crizotinib. Int J Radiat Oncol Biol Phys 2014;88:892–898.

112 Park C, Papiez L, Zhang S, Story M, Timmerman RD: Universal survival curve and single fraction equivalent dose: useful tools in understanding potency of ablative radiotherapy. Int J Radiat Oncol Biol Phys 2008;70:847–852.

113 Folkert MR, Timmerman R: Review of treatment options for oligometastatic non-small cell lung cancer. Clin Adv Hematol Oncol 2015;13:186–193.

114 Tree AC, Khoo VS, Eeles RA, Ahmed M, Dearnaley DP, Hawkins MA, Huddart RA, Nutting CM, Ostler PJ, van As NJ: Stereotactic body radiotherapy for oligometastases. Lancet Oncol 2013;14:e28–e37.

Prof. Dr. Matthias Guckenberger, MD
Department of Radiation Oncology
University Hospital Zurich (USZ)
Rämistrasse 100, CH–8091 Zurich (Switzerland)
E-Mail matthias.guckenberger@usz.ch

Guckenberger M, Combs SE, Zips D (eds): Advances in Radiotherapy.
Prog Tumor Res. Basel, Karger, 2018, vol 44, pp 89–104 (DOI: 10.1159/000486997)

Clinical Rationale and Indications for Particle Therapy

Constantin Dreher · Stephanie E. Combs

Department of Radiation Oncology, Technische Universität München (TUM), Klinikum rechts der Isar, Munich, Germany

Abstract

Particle therapy is characterized by distinct physical properties leading to a reduction of integral dose compared to photons. While protons have an almost comparable biological effect, carbon ions and other heavier charged particles offer an increased relative biological effectiveness. The potential clinical benefit has been pointed out by several groups. Most likely, for protons, children have the largest margin of benefit since their normal tissue is very sensitive to radiation, and curative treatments lead to extremely long-term survivors having a lot of scope for long-term side effects. Many clinical studies, mostly of a retrospective nature, have shown promising results for various tumor types being treated with proton and heavy ion radiotherapy. Further clinical trials are needed in order to evaluate the opportunities of ion beam therapy and its prognostic influence on the general outcome, and many studies are currently recruiting patients. The aim here is to summarize current knowledge, possible clinical rationales, and indications for ion beam therapy. © 2018 S. Karger AG, Basel

Early treatment trials were restricted to tumors that were difficult to irradiate. Due to the physical properties of particle beams, the idea was to increase the dose to the tumor, which is possible due to their dose distributions. Based on the inverted depth-dose curve, the reduction of dose exposure to the normal tissues has mainly been the rationale for the use of ion beam therapy. With promising results in terms of increased dose application and the enhanced radiobiological effectiveness of both protons and heavy ions, the early indications of ion beam therapy were mainly limited to radioresistant tumors. Recently, other tumor types have also begun to be investigated. Generally, the rationale for carbon ions is often seen in radiation-resistant, sometimes slow-growing tumors, such as chordomas. As for protons, indications are set a little wider, focusing on tumor types of various histologies generally with the aim to reduce long-term side effects.

Central Nervous System Tumors

Gliomas and Meningiomas

High-grade glioma and atypical meningioma are characterized by high radioresistance, which is why these tumors may profit most from ion beam therapy. For low-grade tumors, the benefit of a reduction in integral dose has the potential to reduce acute as well as long-term side effects. Therefore, protons have a certain rationale, especially in low-grade gliomas and benign meningiomas. With high-linear energy transfer (LET) particles, such as carbon ions, one may exploit the radiobiological properties of these beams for a potential increase in outcome. This might be a promising concept in high-grade meningiomas as well as high-grade gliomas.

Japanese facilities have produced promising results, showing the superiority of combined photon and carbon ion radiotherapy versus photon radiotherapy alone in patients with WHO III and IV gliomas after resection [1]. On the basis of a retrospective analysis of postoperative combined photon and carbon ion radiotherapy with concurrent temozolomide (demonstrating the potential benefit of this concept), the CLEOPATRA trial with postoperative radiochemotherapy with temozolomide (photon radiotherapy of 50 Gy) followed by a carbon ion (18-Gy relative biological effectiveness [RBE]) versus proton boost (10-Gy [RBE]) at Heidelberger Ion-Beam Therapy Center (HIT) has been set up [2, 3]. Two Japanese trials on combined high-dose photon and proton boost radiotherapy (50.4 + 46.2 Gy [RBE] or 50.4 + 23.1 Gy [RBE] + 23.1 Gy [RBE]) with concurrent temozolomide or nimustine hydrochloride had satisfying 2-year overall survival rates of 45.3% [4, 5].

Besides high-grade gliomas, low-grade gliomas have also been successfully treated with proton radiotherapy of 54 Gy (RBE) with 3- and 5-year progression-free survival rates of 85 and 40% and only few side effects [6, 7]. Hasegawa et al. [8] could also show that overall survival and progression-free survival were higher with carbon ion radiotherapy of 55.2 Gy (RBE) than with smaller doses, while at same time showing acceptable toxicity. A study on pediatric patients with low-grade gliomas could even demonstrate 8-year progression-free survival rates of 82.8% after proton radiotherapy with a median of 52.2 Gy (RBE) [9].

Meningiomas account for about 15% of all primary central nervous system tumors, of which only 10% are atypical ones. The treatment of choice is resection, but skull base and recurrent meningiomas profit from high-dose radiotherapy. In general, photon irradiation with a cumulative dose over 60 Gy leads to satisfactory survival, but there is no advantage of combined photon and proton irradiation over high-dose photon radiotherapy of benign meningiomas in terms of local control rates [10–13]. This may be explained by reduced robustness due to sharp dose gradients or the fact that mainly atypical, skull base, and recurrent meningiomas profit from radiotherapy. However, this is not fully understood and needs to be reevaluated in prospective trials, directly comparing photon and particle radiotherapy. With regard to recurrent and atypical meningiomas, radiotherapy has to be improved in order to increase the local control and overall survival rate. Small trials with photons could show that doses exceeding 60 Gy are required [11]. Dose escalation trials, especially in the case of skull-base tumors, should be conducted by ion beam therapy. Radiotherapy with heavy ions can possibly overcome the results of proton or high-dose photon radiotherapy. On the basis of first results of the Gesellschaft für Schwerionenforschung (GSI) in Germany, a clinical trial of combined photon and carbon ion radiotherapy (50.4 Gy photon radiotherapy + 18 Gy [RBE] carbon ion radiotherapy boost) has been initiated at HIT [14, 15]. To date, proton data are comparable to photons; however, randomized trials are still missing to confirm any superiority.

Skull Base Cancer

Skull-base tumors are characterized by highly radiosensitive normal tissues surrounding the tumor, which is why conformal radiotherapy is of utmost importance. The proximity of tumor and cranial nerves or major vessels results in oncologically incomplete resections with additive radiotherapy afterwards, which is why Fossati et al. [16] concluded that proton radiotherapy plays a major role in skull-base malignancies. Here, especially the potential to dose-escalate is the strongest argument for particles.

Ion beam therapy shows superior results compared to photon irradiation with regard to both dose distribution and clinical results, especially in the case of chordomas and chondrosarcomas [17–22]. The Paul Scherrer Institute (PSI) showed actuarial 5-year local control rates of 81 and 94% after proton radiotherapy of chordomas and chondrosarcomas (73.5 Gy [RBE] and 68.4 Gy [RBE]). At HIT, carbon ion radiotherapy of a median 60 Gy (RBE) leads to local control and overall survival rates of 72 and 75% after 5 years [23]. On top of that, HIT could show the safety and efficacy of reirradiation with carbon ions (51.0 Gy [RBE]) of recurrent skull-base chordomas and chondrosarcomas [24].

Irradiation after surgery is even more important in patients with chordomas, as chordomas frequently recur after incomplete resections. The combination of precise head immobilization, and the physical and the biological characteristics of ion beam therapy allows high-dose applications in the target volume of the skull base. This is important, as a clear dose-response relationship was found in chordoma patients and the local control rate probability improved with a cumulative dose exceeding 60 Gy (RBE) – at least 57.36 Gy (RBE) should be recommended [17, 20, 21, 25, 26]. As described before, PSI showed actuarial 5-year local control rates of 81% after proton radiotherapy with 73.5 Gy (RBE). The GSI showed actuarial 5-year local control rates of only 70% after carbon ion radiotherapy of skull base chordomas with 60

Gy (RBE) [17]. However, the National Institute of Radiological Sciences (NIRS) could show superior local control rates (5-year local control rate of 100%) by the use of carbon ion radiotherapy of up to 60.8 Gy (RBE) in a phase II trial on chordomas [21].

With regard to chondrosarcoma, the ideal therapy has not yet been found, but postoperative high-dose ion beam therapy results in good local control rates in general. At the Massachusetts General Hospital (MGH) in Boston and several other ion beam therapy facilities, 5-year local control rates of 78–99% have been achieved [27–29]. Overall survival rates of 5 and 10 years after adjuvant proton radiotherapy or combined photon and proton radiotherapy with a cumulative dose of 70.2 Gy (RBE) are 94.9 and 87% [29]. These results could be confirmed by the PSI with an 8-year overall survival rate of 93.5% after postoperative proton radiotherapy with a median dose of 70 Gy (RBE) [30]. A differentiated therapy on the basis of grading has not been established, but Pritchard et al. [31] showed its significant influence. At present, HIT is conducting clinical trials comparing proton and carbon ion radiotherapy for patients with chordoma (63 Gy [RBE] vs. 72 Gy [RBE]) and chondrosarcoma (60 Gy [RBE] vs. 70 Gy [RBE]) of the skull base [32, 33].

Sarcoma

There is still little evidence on ion beam radiotherapy in cases of both bone and soft tissue sarcoma. However, there are results from NIRS, showing convincing results for carbon ion radiotherapy of sarcomas in general and especially in cases of head and neck sarcomas [34, 35]. Chordomas are a special entity of sarcomas, but seem to be highly sensitive to carbon ion radiotherapy [36, 37].

Skull base chordomas and chondrosarcomas were discussed above. Evidence is so far limited in the case of chordomas and chondrosarcomas of the spine. Postoperative proton radiotherapy in a small cohort analysis by Holliday et al. [38] was accompanied by high recurrence rates even after the delivery of 70 Gy (RBE). Nevertheless, there are long-term results of proton radiotherapy of 72.4 Gy (RBE) or combined photon and proton radiotherapy of up to 77.4 Gy (RBE) of different spine sarcomas with 5- and 8-year overall survival rates of 81 and 52% [39, 40].

Carbon ion radiotherapy only or combined photon and carbon ion radiotherapy (median 66 Gy [RBE]) of sacrococcygeal chordomas at HIT resulted in a 3-year overall survival rate of 100% with a 3-year local control rate of 53% [41]. Imai et al. [36] could even present results from a cohort of 188 cases of carbon ion radiotherapy (64–73.6 Gy [RBE]) of unresectable sacral chordoma with a 5-year overall survival rate of 81.1%. These results are highly promising. However, definitive results about which kind of sarcoma profits most from which kind of ion beam therapy, the role of primary or recurrent chordoma, and the relation of surgery and ion beam therapy are still lacking.

Head and Neck Cancer

Adenoid cystic carcinoma (ACC) is by far the most radioresistant carcinoma of the group of head and neck cancers showing superior prognostic results by combined ion and photon radiotherapy in contrast to photon radiotherapy alone [42, 43]. In the case of ACC of the skull base, there are very promising results from MGH in Boston with combined photon and proton radiotherapy (cumulative 75.8 Gy [RBE]) after biopsy, partial or total resection, with a 5-year local control rate of 94% [43]. Gentile et al. [44] demonstrated a 5-year overall survival rate of 59% after definitive proton radiotherapy of 73.8 Gy (RBE) in unresectable ACC of the nasopharynx.

At HIT combined photon radiotherapy of 54 Gy followed by carbon ion radiotherapy of up to 18 Gy (RBE) was superior to isolated photon ra-

diotherapy of a median of 66 Gy [45]. A phase III trial with fast neutron radiotherapy compared to photon radiotherapy showed higher 10-year local control rates of 56% with high-LET radiotherapy [46]. Another study by Douglas et al. [47] on fast neutron therapy of ACC resulted in 5-year local control and auctorial overall survival rates of 57 and 72%.

Thus, the poor prognosis of ACC, which is mainly based on perineural extension, is improved by the use of ion beam therapy [48]. There is only little evidence on the comparison of proton and carbon ion radiotherapy in this setting – a Japanese study did not detect any significant difference after 65 Gy (RBE) of proton or carbon ion radiotherapy [49]. On top of that, we have limited knowledge on long-term outcome after ion beam therapy, as late recurrence is common in ACC patients. However, the complication rate is lower with ion beam therapy and carbon ion radiotherapy is even feasible and effective in the case of reirradiation with more than 50 Gy (RBE) [50].

Locally advanced parotid gland carcinoma can be feasibly treated with definitive carbon ion radiotherapy of 64 Gy (RBE), resulting in a 5-year overall survival rate of 70.1% – an important element of this analysis is that a big part of the cohort were ACC patients [51]. Postoperative or definitive combined photon (50 Gy) and carbon ion radiotherapy (24 Gy [RBE]) of malignant salivary gland tumors (COSMIC trial at HIT) resulted in 3-year overall survival and local control rates of 78.4 and 81.9% [52].

Another tumor of interest in patients with head and neck cancer is malignant melanoma. A retrospective study of about 260 patients with mucosal melanoma of the head and neck showed promising results after a median of 57.6 Gy (RBE) carbon ion radiotherapy, although one has to be clear about the fact that half of the patients received concurrent chemotherapy: 2-year overall survival and local control rates were 69.4 and 83.9% [53]. The long-term toxicity seems to be acceptable [54].

Head and neck cancer in general can safely be irradiated by proton beams, but an overall superiority in the case of prognosis could not be shown until now (except for ACC) [55]. Due to the decreased integral dose, toxicity rates are lower for proton than for photon radiotherapy [56]. A multi-institutional review confirmed the feasibility, especially in the case of reirradiation with 60.6 Gy (RBE) proton radiotherapy, of recurrent head and neck cancer [57]. A comparison of carbon ion radiotherapy (median 57.6 Gy [RBE] in 16 fractions) and Cyberknife radiotherapy (35 Gy in 5 fractions) could even show higher survival rates in the case of ion beam reirradiation of recurrent head and neck cancer [58]. The combination of reirradiation with protons and chemotherapy might lead to an even more advantageous outcome [59].

Lung Cancer

Lung cancer is associated with the highest rate of cancer deaths worldwide [60]. Developments of precise dose delivery in moving cancers, such as tracking, gating, and stereotactic body radiotherapy (SBRT) led to an increase in the use of radiotherapy in lung cancers. Nevertheless, radiotherapy needs to achieve a further reduction of dose application to the surrounding normal tissues and has to improve local control rates. A retrospective analysis by Higgins et al. [61] of non-small-cell lung cancer (NSCLC) in general showed a superior outcome after proton radiotherapy compared to photon radiotherapy.

Early-Stage NSCLC

In general, surgery is the preferred choice of treatment in early-stage NSCLC. It leads to a 5-year survival rate of over 60%, in contrast to about 30% with conventional, fractionated radiotherapy [62–64]. This is the reason why further improvement in radiotherapy is required. SBRT could prove its efficacy in the case of NSCLC, but there are studies promoting the role of proton radiotherapy with 4-year overall survival rates of 70 and 16% in IA and IB stage NSCLC [65–67]. Bush et al. [68] reported results of combined photon and proton radiotherapy in stage IA and IB NSCLC with 3-year disease-specific survival rates of 74 and 72%. To date, Bush et al. [69] have established a hypofractionated proton radiotherapy concept of 70 Gy (RBE) in 10 fractions for T1-2 N0M0 NSCLC. Nakayama et al. [70] and Hatayama et al. [71] showed 3-year progression-free survival rates of 76.3 and 79% after proton radiotherapy with 66 Gy (RBE) or 72.6 Gy (RBE) in peripheral and central, inoperable stage I NSCLC. Chang et al. [72] showed a 5-year overall survival rate of 28.1% after 87.5 Gy (RBE) proton radiotherapy in inoperable early-stage NSCLC.

These results of proton radiotherapy are highly promising, but there is still little evidence of high-LET radiotherapy, and there is no direct, prospective comparison of different ion beam therapy concepts. Nevertheless, based on the results after proton radiotherapy, carbon ion radiotherapy seems to be appropriate in early-stage NSCLC and can potentially exceed these results, as hypofractionated carbon ion radiotherapy (72 Gy RBE) in 9 fractions or (52.8 Gy [RBE]) in 4 fractions of stage I NSCLC leads to 5-year overall survival rates of 45–50% [73, 74]. A single-fraction dose-escalation trial could even prove its feasibility and efficacy with 5-year overall survival rates of 69.2% after 48–50 Gy (RBE) of carbon ion irradiation [75].

However, a retrospective comparison of proton and carbon ion radiotherapy (52.8–80.0 Gy [RBE] and 52.8–70.2 Gy [RBE]) could not detect a superiority of one kind of ion beam therapy in stage I NSCLC [76].

Advanced-Stage NSCLC

Complete resection is the treatment of choice, but in many situations surgery is not possible. Radiotherapy in advanced-stage NSCLC is mainly performed in stage IIIB, although associated with a poor prognosis. Modern radiotherapy techniques with photons and in stage III simultaneous chemotherapy is the standard treatment if surgery is not possible [77–79].

The prognosis is generally poor and with the use of proton radiotherapy we have to rely on trials with very small patient numbers. A dose-escalation study by Harada et al. [80] concluded that a cumulative dose of 66 Gy (RBE) of proton radiotherapy should be the recommended dose in stage III NSCLC. Shioyama et al. [65] reported 2-year overall survival rates of 62%, and Nguyen et al. [81] published 3-year overall survival rates of 41–52% depending on the stage.

Takahashi et al. [82] reported 2-year overall survival rates after 68–76 Gy (RBE) carbon ion radiotherapy of 51.9%. Nevertheless, particle therapy should be associated with a better prognosis, as it allows the deposition of higher doses in the target volume and decreased dose exposure of the surrounding normal tissue. Therefore, the PRONTOX trial aims to prove the decreased rate of side effects of proton radiotherapy compared to photon radiotherapy of advanced-stage NSCLC [83].

Ion beam therapy in general could demonstrate its feasibility but, similar to the irradiation of liver cancer robustness, there is the major problem of lung cancer irradiation. With the lung being a highly mobile organ, precise dose delivery is of utmost importance. Ion beam therapy, especially by the use of the raster scanning technique, needs to overcome this problem, as the risk of interplay affects increases [84, 85]. However, compensating for the decrease of robustness by the use of tracking and gating, together with the radiobiological opportunities of carbon ion radiotherapy, are highly promising, and randomized trials have to be conducted [84, 86]. At NIRS, the feasibility of scattered carbon ion radiotherapy on the basis of image guidance by the use of fiducial markers, immobilization by the use of thermoplastic plates, and gating by the use of position-sensitive detectors could be demonstrated [87].

Liver and Pancreatic Cancer

Hepatocellular Carcinoma

Hepatocellular carcinoma (HCC) is a challenging entity of cancer. Globally, HCC is the third leading cause of cancer death [88]. Early-stage HCC is treated either by surgical resection or liver transplantation, but most patients are ineligible for surgery, thus leading to therapy options that aim to bridge to transplantation or can be used in palliative therapy. With technological advances, stereotactic radiotherapy is an important option in the treatment of selected HCC patients [89]. Nevertheless, locoregional procedures still present a poor prognosis, which is why treatment options such as the well-established SBRT have to be improved. As HCC is mainly based on hepatitis B, C, or alcoholic cirrhosis with subsequent impaired liver function, and these patients have an even lower tolerance of radiation to the liver, possibly resulting in radiotherapy-induced liver disease [90–92]. However, with the actual dose being predictive for tumor control, radiation techniques have to aim at enabling an increasing radiation dose to the tumor [93, 94]. Ion beam therapy is able to increase the applied dose in the tumor and to preserve the surrounding liver tissue, thus resulting in less toxicity compared to high-precision stereotactic radiotherapy and at the same time being characterized by similar or superior survival rates [95]. However, the highly localized dose escalation in the liver is very difficult, as robustness in the breathing-induced liver motion is of utmost importance. Ion beam therapy, especially scanned ion beam therapy, has to be critically evaluated. The placement of fiducial markers is recommended for image-guided radiotherapy, both with photons and particles [96]. Fractionated ion beam therapy is able to reduce dose inhomogeneity by interplay effects, but robust treatment planning is still the major problem of precise dose delivery in ion beam therapy of liver malignancies [97].

Nevertheless, Hata et al. [98] and Kato et al. [99] achieved highly promising results with carbon ion and proton radiotherapy of HCC, which is why further investigations and the clinical rationale have to be analyzed. Proton radiotherapy with doses beginning at 60 Gy (RBE) have to be applied, but liver function and pretreatments must be included in the decision process. Nakayama et al. [100] showed a 5-year overall actuarial survival rate of 44.6% after proton radiotherapy. Bush et al. [101, 102] demonstrated a 2-year overall survival rate of 55% and 3-year progression-free survival of 60% after proton radiotherapy with 63 Gy (RBE) with very few adverse side effects. The 2-year overall survival and local control rates in a prospective phase II trial of hypofractionated proton radiotherapy of unresectable HCC with a median of 58 Gy (RBE) were 63.2 and 94.8% [103]. Interim analysis from Bush et al. [104] of a prospective comparison of TACE versus proton radiotherapy of 70.2 Gy (RBE) showed similar survival rates with a trend of improved local control rate by proton radiotherapy. Sugahara et al. [105, 106] and Kimura et al. [107] could demonstrate the feasibility of proton radiotherapy in large HCC volumes and HCC with portal vein thrombosis. On top of that, proton radiotherapy seems to be beneficial, especially in the case of tumor vessel thrombosis [108, 109]. Oshiro et al. [110] could also show that repeated proton radiotherapy of HCC with a median of 70.5 Gy (RBE) is characterized by good overall survival rates and few side effects, even in the case of mean doses to the liver exceeding critical dose constraints of radiotherapy-induced liver disease. Thus, there are clinical results showing the feasibility of proton radiotherapy under difficult conditions, but it is still unclear which patients profit most from ion beam therapy. Japanese results are also based on highly hypofractionated dose regimes, demonstrating the feasibility of ion beam application and the relatively limited treatment-associated side effects.

The dose-escalation trial PROMETHEUS-01 at HIT aims to analyze the rationale of raster-scanned carbon ion radiotherapy in HCC patients. However, long-term results are not available yet [111].

Pancreatic Cancer
Pancreatic cancer patients have a poor prognosis, with 277,000 deaths worldwide recorded each year due to this disease [112]. Resection is considered to be the only curative treatment, but in cases of locally advanced unresectable pancreatic cancer (LAPC), neoadjuvant treatment approaches such as combined chemoradiation or chemotherapy lead to downstaging with secondary resectability in approximately 30% [113–117]. However, ion beam therapy with its inverted depth-dose curve may be appropriate, especially in pancreatic malignancies, where radiosensitive organs such as the stomach, liver, and kidneys surround the target volume [118–120]. The main organ at risk in ion beam therapy of pancreatic cancer is the stomach/small bowel, thus leading to radiation-induced ulcers in up to 50% of patients after proton radiotherapy with concurrent gemcitabine application [121].

Despite the high risk of radiation-induced side effects, combined proton radiotherapy of 50 Gy (RBE) with concurrent gemcitabine is generally well tolerated, similarly to proton radiotherapy of 50.4–59.4 Gy (RBE) with concurrent capecitabine [122, 123]. Furthermore, preoperative short-course chemoradiotherapy with proton beams (25 Gy [RBE] in 5 fractions) and capecitabine could prove its feasibility in resectable pancreatic cancer [124].

Carbon ion beams in particular offer a higher biological effectiveness compared to proton beams, which might further increase the resectability of LAPC and decrease radiation-induced side effects [125–127]. There are encouraging clinical results with hypofractionated carbon ion radiotherapy of up to 55.2 Gy (RBE) and concurrent gemcitabine of LAPC [119, 128, 129]. A phase I trial of preoperative short-course carbon ion radiotherapy of up to 36.8 Gy (RBE) in patients with resectable pancreatic cancer resulted in promising 5-year overall survival rates of 42 and 52% for patients with and without surgery after radiotherapy [119]. Nevertheless, despite their pressing need, to date there are no clinical trials directly comparing proton and carbon ion radiotherapy in pancreatic cancer patients.

Gastrointestinal Cancer

Esophagus Cancer

If resectable, surgery is the current treatment of choice for esophagus cancer. Otherwise, definitive or neoadjuvant simultaneous radiochemotherapy are recommended, depending on the localization and the stage of the tumor.

To date, there is still little evidence on the role of particle therapy, but there are promising results, especially from Japanese and American institutions. Locally advanced esophageal cancer has been treated with combined photon and proton radiotherapy (median cumulative dose of 80 Gy [RBE]) resulting in promising 5-year local control rates of 38% [130]. Combined proton radiotherapy (60 Gy [RBE]) and chemotherapy with cisplatin/5-fluoruracil was also feasible – the locoregional control rate was 66% after 2 years and overall survival rate was 70% after 3 years [131]. Lin et al. [132] showed encouraging results of preoperative and definitive combined proton radiotherapy (median 50.4 Gy [RBE]) and chemotherapy with an estimated 3-year overall survival rate of 52%.

Similarly, a phase I/II trial on preoperative short-course carbon ion radiotherapy of up to 36.8 Gy (RBE) in squamous cell carcinoma of the esophagus resulted in a 38.7% complete response and 61% 5-year overall survival rate [133]. These results are encouraging, but results based on prospective trials about particle beam radiotherapy of esophageal cancer are of utmost importance.

Rectal Cancer

Surgical resection of rectal cancer, especially in the case of advanced-stage rectal cancer, should be accompanied by preoperative or postoperative radiochemotherapy. Preoperative radiochemotherapy can lead to significant downstaging and reduces local failure rates [134]. In the case of recurrent rectal cancer, therapeutic options are limited and prognosis is still poor. Ion beam therapy might be one option. The first Japanese results could show local control rates of up to 81.3% at 3 years after hypofractionated carbon ion radiotherapy with 67.2–73.6 Gy (RBE) [135]. Five years after carbon ion radiotherapy with 73.6 Gy (RBE) in patients with recurrent rectal cancer, local control and overall survival rates were 88 and 59%, respectively [136]. These results are highly promising and further prospective trials are needed.

Prostate Cancer

In male patients, prostate cancer is the major cancer with the highest incidence [60]. Surgery and radiotherapy are the major treatment options and radiotherapy, especially in early-stage prostate cancer, is characterized by a good prognosis and only few side effects. The topic of current studies is consequently the reduction of all side effects. Due to the reduction of dose exposure to the surrounding normal tissues, ion beam therapy is very attractive. On top of that, prostate cancer is characterized by a very low α/β ratio, thus leading to a theoretical superiority of ion beam therapy, and especially hypofractionated ion beam therapy, over photon radiotherapy [137].

The first results at MGH and Loma Linda University Medical Center showed promising results in combined photon and proton radiotherapy and isolated proton radiotherapy [138–140]. In subsequent trials, no superiority of proton radiotherapy in overall survival could be detected, but a benefit in side effects with little toxicity could be shown [141–145]. With prostate cancer being characterized by a low α/β ratio, trials on hypofractionated proton radiotherapy are conducted with the first results demonstrating its feasibility and safety [146, 147]. However, due to the limited proven superiority, questions arise as to whether ion beam therapy and especially proton radiotherapy is really as beneficial as presumed [148]. In contrast to these questions, recent results about proton radiotherapy with 78 Gy (RBE) in patients with localized prostate cancer resulted in excellent survival rates and low rates of high-grade toxicity [149].

Carbon ion radiotherapy might even exceed the results of proton radiotherapy of prostate cancer. The first trials on hypofractionated carbon ion radiotherapy of 54–72 Gy (RBE) for patients with early-stage and locally advanced prostate cancer revealed a 5-year overall survival rate of 89.2% with little morbidity [150]. A multi-institutional analysis of prospective studies with hypofractionated carbon ion radiotherapy of 51.6–66 Gy (RBE) in 12–20 fractions showed favorable results with 10-year overall survival rates of 96, 78, and 88% for low, intermediate, and high-risk patients [151]. Hypofractionation in carbon ion radiotherapy was not associated with a higher risk of toxicity [152]. Generally, morbidity in carbon ion radiotherapy of prostate cancer is mainly based on gastrointestinal toxicity, which is why Rucinski et al. [153] at HIT introduced the dosimetric benefit of a spacer gel in ion beam therapy.

Further investigations on the radiobiological characteristics of prostate cancer are needed, and carbon ion beam irradiation in prostate cancer might be the one therapy that improves the prognosis of prostate cancer patients while further reducing side effects of photon radiotherapy [150, 154–157]. On top of that, the role of androgen deprivation prior to or after radiotherapy has not yet been evaluated, which is why future trials need to take this into account. The possible advantages of ion beam therapy are reduced rectal toxicity and a potential reduction of secondary cancer after radiotherapy. This needs to be addressed as well.

Gynecological Malignancies

Radiotherapy of gynecological malignancies in the pelvis is mainly based on radiotherapy combined with intracavitary brachytherapy, locally applying high doses with a sharp gradient and resulting in good local control rates. Simultaneous application of chemotherapy is often beneficial in the case of locally advanced stages with 5-year local control and overall survival rates of 56–71 and 67–80% in stage III-IVA [158]. Nevertheless, local failure and side effects by combined radiochemotherapy still call for improvements in current standard treatment options [158, 159].

Only small clinical trials about proton radiotherapy of cervical cancer have been conducted at the Tsukuba University. Kagei et al. [160] demonstrated 5-year overall survival rates of 40–89% of a heterogeneous group of stage IIB-IVA cervical cancer patients treated with different regimes of combined photon and proton radiotherapy.

Carbon ion radiotherapy of stage IIIB-IVA patients with cervical cancer resulted in a cumulative 2-year survival rate of 61.5% in the dose escalation trial [161, 162]. Side effects were mainly based on high-dose application over 60 Gy (RBE) in the adjacent GI tract, although generally with favorable local tumor control rates. Recent results in carbon ion radiotherapy of stage IIB-IVA showed 5-year local control and overall survival rates of 54.5 and 38.1% [163]. A meta-analysis of locally advanced cervical cancer with bladder invasion showed 3-year local control and overall survival rates of 66 and 47% [164].

Therefore, in summary, there is only little evidence on ion beam therapy and the results until now do not show high superiority of ion beam radiotherapy over photon radiotherapy. On top of that, precise dose delivery is again a major problem, as different bladder and rectal fillings can cause a systematic error, especially in the case of sharp dose gradients with ion beam radiotherapy [165].

Pediatric Cancer

Ion beam therapy in pediatric patients is of special interest, as the integral dose is reduced compared to photon radiotherapy, thus leading to a potentially decreased risk of secondary carcinoma [166–168]. On top of that, with the treatment options developing over time, the cure rate of pediatric cancer patients has increased as well, which is why late morbidity has to be decreased in order to ensure quality of life [169, 170]. Nonmalignant late side effects in pediatrics are organ dysfunctions, such as neurocognitive impairment, sterility, and growth inhibition or dysfunction. Consequently, dose exposure to normal tissue has to be reduced as far as possible.

Craniospinal irradiation with protons has been successfully established with a lower incidence of organ-at-risk dysfunction, but similar overall survival [171–173]. The advantage of ion beam therapy over photon radiotherapy is radiation protection, which is why proton radiotherapy of brain tumors leads to higher intelligence quotients than photon radiotherapy [174].

Carbon ion radiotherapy has to be critically evaluated. It might be advantageous in cases of hypoxic or radioresistant tumors, such as sarcoma, but the dose distribution is different from proton radiotherapy. Carbon ion radiotherapy is superior to proton radiotherapy in terms of lateral dose gradients, but inferior with regard to dose exposure distal of the so-called Bragg peak.

In general, there is little evidence on particle therapy of children, but trials are ongoing aiming at identifying the situations in which ion beam therapy might be superior to photon radiotherapy. Especially in the case of brain or head and neck tumors, several studies have shown the feasibility and efficacy of proton beam therapy in pediatric patients.

Medulloblastomas are treated with resection of the primary tumor and afterwards craniospinal irradiation with proton radiotherapy of 18–36 Gy (RBE) and a following boost of up to 54 Gy (RBE) at best [175, 176]. Proton radiotherapy leads to overall survival rates similar to photon radiotherapy (5-year overall survival rate of 83%), but is associated with low rates of toxicity and can even reduce some of the risks of radiation-associated late endocrine abnormalities [176, 177].

Craniopharyngioma, ependymoma, and rhabdomyosarcoma have already been treated with proton radiotherapy [178–180]. Craniopharyngioma can hardly be totally resected, which is why radiotherapy is of utmost importance. Luu et al. [178] and Laffond et al. [181] demonstrated the possible use of proton radiotherapy (50.4–59.4 Gy [RBE]), and its high impact on the quality of life of children with the decreased dose exposure to the surrounding normal tissues [178, 181]. Nevertheless, in review of current evidence, no significant difference in survival rates and toxicity between photon and proton radiotherapy could be detected [182].

Ependymoma are generally resected and locally irradiated afterwards. Small trials could demonstrate both the feasibility of proton radiotherapy (50.4–61.2 Gy [RBE]) even in the case of reirradiation and dosimetric superiority with regard to neurologic functioning [179, 183–186].

Rhabdomyosarcomas are very radioresistant, but proton radiotherapy seems to be feasible, although accompanied by high morbidity (nevertheless, still lower than with photon radiotherapy) [187, 188]. Ladra et al. [189] published preliminary results of a phase-II trial of proton radiotherapy (median 50.4 Gy [RBE]) with concurrent chemotherapy with fewer radiation-induced side effects compared to photon radiotherapy. However, the still existing high local failure rate is probably not due to the sharp dosimetric gradients, thus leading to the question of how to improve therapy of rhabdomyosarcoma [190]. In contrast, Leiser et al. [191] showed excellent results with 5-year local control rates of 78.5% after proton radiotherapy of 54 Gy (RBE) of rhabdomyosarcoma with little morbidity.

There are several other possible indications of ion beam radiotherapy in pediatric malignancies, but we have to conclude that there is only little evidence of the effect of ion beam therapy (especially high-LET radiotherapy) on patient outcome. Nevertheless, ion beam radiotherapy is highly promising, which is why we are in desperate need of prospective trials, especially in pediatric malignancies.

Conclusion

Ion beam therapy represents one of the main improvements in radiation oncology in recent years. Unfortunately, there are still only a few facilities offering ion beam therapy. A distinction must be made between protons, where indications can be considered comparable to photons, and high-LET particle beams, where clinical trials are necessary due to the intricate biological differences. In recent years, the number of proton radiotherapy facilities has increased, but the number of carbon ion radiotherapy facilities is still very limited. With availability being so restricted, and basic and clinical research still being at an early stage, we have to conduct new trials evaluating the pros and cons of ion beam therapy, which will finally lead to better patient care.

References

1 Mizoe JE, et al: Phase I/II clinical trial of carbon ion radiotherapy for malignant gliomas: combined X-ray radiotherapy, chemotherapy, and carbon ion radiotherapy. Int J Radiat Oncol Biol Phys 2007;69:390–396.

2 Combs SE, et al: Comparison of carbon ion radiotherapy to photon radiation alone or in combination with temozolomide in patients with high-grade gliomas: explorative hypothesis-generating retrospective analysis. Radiother Oncol 2013;108:132–135.

3 Combs SE, et al: Randomized phase II study evaluating a carbon ion boost applied after combined radiochemotherapy with temozolomide versus a proton boost after radiochemotherapy with temozolomide in patients with primary glioblastoma: the CLEOPATRA trial. BMC Cancer 2010;10:478.

4 Mizumoto M, et al: Phase I/II trial of hyperfractionated concomitant boost proton radiotherapy for supratentorial glioblastoma multiforme. Int J Radiat Oncol Biol Phys 2010;77:98–105.

5 Mizumoto M, et al: Long-term survival after treatment of glioblastoma multiforme with hyperfractionated concomitant boost proton beam therapy. Pract Radiat Oncol 2015;5:e9–e16.

6 Shih HA, et al: Proton therapy for low-grade gliomas: results from a prospective trial. Cancer 2015;121:1712–1719.

7 Hauswald H, et al: First experiences in treatment of low-grade glioma grade I and II with proton therapy. Radiat Oncol 2012;7:189.

8 Hasegawa A, et al: Experience with carbon ion radiotherapy for WHO grade 2 diffuse astrocytomas. Int J Radiat Oncol Biol Phys 2012;83:100–106.

9 Greenberger BA, et al: Clinical outcomes and late endocrine, neurocognitive, and visual profiles of proton radiation for pediatric low-grade gliomas. Int J Radiat Oncol Biol Phys 2014;89:1060–1068.

10 Boskos C, et al: Combined proton and photon conformal radiotherapy for intracranial atypical and malignant meningioma. Int J Radiat Oncol Biol Phys 2009;75:399–406.

11 Hug EB, et al: Management of atypical and malignant meningiomas: role of high-dose, 3D-conformal radiation therapy. J Neurooncol 2000;48:151–160.

12 Noel G, et al: Functional outcome of patients with benign meningioma treated by 3D conformal irradiation with a combination of photons and protons. Int J Radiat Oncol Biol Phys 2005;62: 1412–1422.

13 Vernimmen FJ, et al: Stereotactic proton beam therapy of skull base meningiomas. Int J Radiat Oncol Biol Phys 2001; 49:99–105.

14 Combs SE, et al: Treatment of patients with atypical meningiomas Simpson grade 4 and 5 with a carbon ion boost in combination with postoperative photon radiotherapy: the MARCIE trial. BMC Cancer 2010;10:615.

15 Combs SE, et al: Carbon ion radiation therapy for high-risk meningiomas. Radiother Oncol 2010;95:54–59.

16 Fossati P, et al: Review of photon and proton radiotherapy for skull base tumours. Rep Pract Oncol Radiother 2016; 21:336–355.

17 Schulz-Ertner D, et al: Effectiveness of carbon ion radiotherapy in the treatment of skull-base chordomas. Int J Radiat Oncol Biol Phys 2007;68:449–457.

18 Schulz-Ertner D, et al: Carbon ion radiotherapy of skull base chondrosarcomas.
Int J Radiat Oncol Biol Phys 2007;67:
171–177.

19 Fuller DB, Bloom JG: Radiotherapy for
chordoma. Int J Radiat Oncol Biol Phys
1988;15:331–339.

20 Mizoe JE: Review of carbon ion radiotherapy for skull base tumors (especially
chordomas). Rep Pract Oncol Radiother
2016;21:356–360.

21 Mizoe JE, et al: Carbon ion radiotherapy
for skull base chordoma. Skull Base
2009;19:219–224.

22 Ares C, et al: Effectiveness and safety of
spot scanning proton radiation therapy
for chordomas and chondrosarcomas of
the skull base: first long-term report. Int
J Radiat Oncol Biol Phys 2009;75:1111–
1118.

23 Uhl M, et al: Highly effective treatment
of skull base chordoma with carbon ion
irradiation using a raster scan technique
in 155 patients: first long-term results.
Cancer 2014;120:3410–3417.

24 Uhl M, et al: Active raster scanning with
carbon ions: reirradiation in patients
with recurrent skull base chordomas
and chondrosarcomas. Strahlenther
Onkol 2014;190:686–691.

25 Tai PT, Craighead P, Bagdon F: Optimization of radiotherapy for patients with
cranial chordoma: a review of dose-response ratios for photon techniques.
Cancer 1995;75:749–756.

26 Matloob SA, Nasir HA, Choi D: Proton
beam therapy in the management of
skull base chordomas: systematic review
of indications, outcomes, and implications for neurosurgeons. Br J Neurosurg
2016;30:382–387.

27 Castro JR, et al: Experience in charged
particle irradiation of tumors of the
skull base: 1977–1992. Int J Radiat Oncol Biol Phys 1994;29:647–655.

28 Rosenberg AE, et al: Chondrosarcoma of
the base of the skull: a clinicopathologic
study of 200 cases with emphasis on its
distinction from chordoma. Am J Surg
Pathol 1999;23:1370–1378.

29 Feuvret L, et al: Efficacy and safety of
adjuvant proton therapy combined with
surgery for chondrosarcoma of the skull
base: a retrospective, population-based
study. Int J Radiat Oncol Biol Phys 2016;
95:312–321.

30 Weber DC, et al: Long-term outcomes
and prognostic factors of skull-base
chondrosarcoma patients treated with
pencil-beam scanning proton therapy at
the Paul Scherrer Institute. Neuro Oncol
2016;18:236–243.

31 Pritchard DJ, et al: Chondrosarcoma: a
clinicopathologic and statistical analysis.
Cancer 1980;45:149–157.

32 Nikoghosyan AV, et al: Randomised
trial of proton vs. carbon ion radiation
therapy in patients with chordoma of
the skull base, clinical phase III study
HIT-1-study. BMC Cancer 2010;10:607.

33 Nikoghosyan AV, et al: Randomised
trial of proton vs. carbon ion radiation
therapy in patients with low and intermediate grade chondrosarcoma of the
skull base, clinical phase III study. BMC
Cancer 2010;10:606.

34 Kamada T, et al: Efficacy and safety of
carbon ion radiotherapy in bone and
soft tissue sarcomas. J Clin Oncol 2002;
20:4466–4471.

35 Jingu K, et al: Carbon ion radiation therapy improves the prognosis of unresectable adult bone and soft-tissue sarcoma
of the head and neck. Int J Radiat Oncol
Biol Phys 2012;82:2125–2131.

36 Imai R, Kamada T, Araki N: Carbon ion
radiation therapy for unresectable sacral
chordoma: an analysis of 188 cases. Int J
Radiat Oncol Biol Phys 2016;95:322–
327.

37 Imai R, et al: Carbon ion radiotherapy
for sacral chordoma. Br J Radiol 2011;
84:S48–S54.

38 Holliday EB, et al: Postoperative proton
therapy for chordomas and chondrosarcomas of the spine: adjuvant versus salvage radiation therapy. Spine 2015;40:
544–549.

39 DeLaney TF, et al: Long-term results of
phase II study of high dose photon/pro-
ton radiotherapy in the management of
spine chordomas, chondrosarcomas,
and other sarcomas. J Surg Oncol 2014;
110:115–122.

40 Rotondo RL, et al: High-dose proton-
based radiation therapy in the management of spine chordomas: outcomes and
clinicopathological prognostic factors. J
Neurosurg Spine 2015;23:788–797.

41 Uhl M, et al: Carbon ion beam treatment
in patients with primary and recurrent
sacrococcygeal chordoma. Strahlenther
Onkol 2015;191:597–603.

42 Jensen AD, et al: High-LET radiotherapy
for adenoid cystic carcinoma of the head
and neck: 15 years’ experience with raster-scanned carbon ion therapy. Radiother Oncol 2016;118:272–280.

43 Pommier P, et al: Proton beam radiation
therapy for skull base adenoid cystic
carcinoma. Arch Otolaryngol Head Neck
Surg 2006;132:1242–1249.

44 Gentile MS, et al: Definitive proton
beam therapy for adenoid cystic carcinoma of the nasopharynx involving the
base of skull. Oral Oncol 2017;65:38–44.

45 Jensen AD, et al: Combined intensity-
modulated radiotherapy plus raster-
scanned carbon ion boost for advanced
adenoid cystic carcinoma of the head
and neck results in superior locoregional control and overall survival. Cancer
2015;121:3001–3009.

46 Laramore GE, et al: Neutron versus photon irradiation for unresectable salivary
gland tumors: final report of an RTOG-
MRC randomized clinical trial. Int J Radiat Oncol Biol Phys 1993;27:235–240.

47 Douglas JG, et al: Treatment of locally
advanced adenoid cystic carcinoma of
the head and neck with neutron radiotherapy. Int J Radiat Oncol Biol Phys
2000;46:551–557.

48 Mendenhall WM, et al: Definitive radiotherapy for skin and adenoid cystic carcinoma with perineural invasion. J Neu-
rol Surg B Skull Base 2016;77:169–172.

49 Takagi M, et al: Treatment outcomes of
particle radiotherapy using protons or
carbon ions as a single-modality therapy
for adenoid cystic carcinoma of the head
and neck. Radiother Oncol 2014;113:
364–370.

50 Jensen AD, et al: Re-irradiation of adenoid cystic carcinoma: analysis and
evaluation of outcome in 52 consecutive
patients treated with raster-scanned
carbon ion therapy. Radiother Oncol
2015;114:182–188.

51 Koto M, et al: Definitive carbon-ion radiotherapy for locally advanced parotid
gland carcinomas. Head Neck 2017;39:
724–729.

52 Jensen AD, et al: COSMIC: a regimen of
intensity modulated radiation therapy
plus dose-escalated, raster-scanned carbon ion boost for malignant salivary
gland tumors: results of the prospective
phase 2 trial. Int J Radiat Oncol Biol
Phys 2015;93:37–46.

53 Koto M, et al: Multicenter study of carbon-ion radiation therapy for mucosal melanoma of the head and neck: sub-analysis of the Japan Carbon-Ion Radiation Oncology Study Group (J-CROS) Study (1402 HN). Int J Radiat Oncol Biol Phys 2017;97:1054–1060.

54 Naganawa K, et al: Long-term outcomes after carbon-ion radiotherapy for oral mucosal malignant melanoma. J Radiat Res 2017;58:517–522.

55 Ramaekers BL, et al: Systematic review and meta-analysis of radiotherapy in various head and neck cancers: comparing photons, carbon-ions and protons. Cancer Treat Rev 2011;37:185–201.

56 Sio TT, et al: Intensity modulated proton therapy versus intensity modulated photon radiation therapy for oropharyngeal cancer: first comparative results of patient-reported outcomes. Int J Radiat Oncol Biol Phys 2016;95:1107–1114.

57 Romesser PB, et al: Proton beam reirradiation for recurrent head and neck cancer: multi-institutional report on feasibility and early outcomes. Int J Radiat Oncol Biol Phys 2016;95:386–395.

58 Yamazaki H, et al: Comparison of re-irradiation outcomes for charged particle radiotherapy and robotic stereotactic radiotherapy using cyberknife for recurrent head and neck cancers: a multi-institutional matched-cohort analysis. Anticancer Res 2016;36:5507–5514.

59 Hayashi Y, et al: Re-irradiation using proton beam therapy combined with weekly intra-arterial chemotherapy for recurrent oral cancer. Asia Pac J Clin Oncol 2017;13:e394–e401.

60 Siegel RL, Miller KD, Jemal A: Cancer statistics, 2017. CA Cancer J Clin 2017; 67:7–30.

61 Higgins KA, et al: National cancer database analysis of proton versus photon radiation therapy in non-small cell lung cancer. Int J Radiat Oncol Biol Phys 2017;97:128–137.

62 Dosoretz DE, et al: Radiation therapy in the management of medically inoperable carcinoma of the lung: results and implications for future treatment strategies. Int J Radiat Oncol Biol Phys 1992; 24:3–9.

63 Sibley GS: Radiotherapy for patients with medically inoperable stage I nonsmall cell lung carcinoma: smaller volumes and higher doses – a review. Cancer 1998;82:433–438.

64 van Rens MT, et al: Prognostic assessment of 2,361 patients who underwent pulmonary resection for non-small cell lung cancer, stage I, II, and IIIA. Chest 2000;117:374–379.

65 Shioyama Y, et al: Clinical evaluation of proton radiotherapy for non-small-cell lung cancer. Int J Radiat Oncol Biol Phys 2003;56:7–13.

66 Blomgren H, et al: Stereotactic high dose fraction radiation therapy of extracranial tumors using an accelerator: clinical experience of the first thirty-one patients. Acta Oncol 1995;34:861–870.

67 McGarry RC, et al: Stereotactic body radiation therapy of early-stage non-small-cell lung carcinoma: phase I study. Int J Radiat Oncol Biol Phys 2005; 63:1010–1015.

68 Bush DA, et al: Hypofractionated proton beam radiotherapy for stage I lung cancer. Chest 2004;126:1198–1203.

69 Bush DA, et al: High-dose hypofractionated proton beam radiation therapy is safe and effective for central and peripheral early-stage non-small cell lung cancer: results of a 12-year experience at Loma Linda University Medical Center. Int J Radiat Oncol Biol Phys 2013;86: 964–968.

70 Nakayama H, et al: Proton beam therapy for patients with medically inoperable stage I non-small-cell lung cancer at the University of Tsukuba. Int J Radiat Oncol Biol Phys 2010;78:467–471.

71 Hatayama Y, et al: Clinical outcomes and prognostic factors of high-dose proton beam therapy for peripheral stage I non-small-cell lung cancer. Clin Lung Cancer 2016;17:427–432.

72 Chang JY, et al: Long-term outcome of phase I/II prospective study of dose-escalated proton therapy for early-stage non-small cell lung cancer. Radiother Oncol 2017;122:274–280.

73 Miyamoto T, et al: Curative treatment of stage I non-small-cell lung cancer with carbon ion beams using a hypofractionated regimen. Int J Radiat Oncol Biol Phys 2007;67:750–758.

74 Miyamoto T, et al: Carbon ion radiotherapy for stage I non-small cell lung cancer using a regimen of four fractions during 1 week. J Thorac Oncol 2007;2: 916–926.

75 Yamamoto N, et al: A dose escalation clinical trial of single-fraction carbon ion radiotherapy for peripheral stage I non-small cell lung cancer. J Thorac Oncol 2017;12:673–680.

76 Fujii O, et al: A retrospective comparison of proton therapy and carbon ion therapy for stage I non-small cell lung cancer. Radiother Oncol 2013;109:32–37.

77 Rosenman JG, et al: High-dose conformal radiotherapy for treatment of stage IIIA/IIIB non-small-cell lung cancer: technical issues and results of a phase I/ II trial. Int J Radiat Oncol Biol Phys 2002;54:348–356.

78 Schild SE, et al: Results of a phase I trial of concurrent chemotherapy and escalating doses of radiation for unresectable non-small-cell lung cancer. Int J Radiat Oncol Biol Phys 2006;65:1106–1111.

79 Socinski MA, et al: Randomized phase II trial of induction chemotherapy followed by concurrent chemotherapy and dose-escalated thoracic conformal radiotherapy (74 Gy) in stage III non-small-cell lung cancer: CALGB 30105. J Clin Oncol 2008;26:2457–2463.

80 Harada H, et al: Dose escalation study of proton beam therapy with concurrent chemotherapy for stage III non-small cell lung cancer. Cancer Sci 2016;107: 1018–1021.

81 Nguyen QN, et al: Long-term outcomes after proton therapy, with concurrent chemotherapy, for stage II-III inoperable non-small cell lung cancer. Radiother Oncol 2015;115:367–372.

82 Takahashi W, et al: A prospective nonrandomized phase I/II study of carbon ion radiotherapy in a favorable subset of locally advanced non-small cell lung cancer (NSCLC). Cancer 2015;121: 1321–1327.

83 Zschaeck S, et al: PRONTOX – proton therapy to reduce acute normal tissue toxicity in locally advanced non-small-cell lung carcinomas (NSCLC): study protocol for a randomised controlled trial. Trials 2016;17:543.

84 Bert C, et al: Gated irradiation with scanned particle beams. Int J Radiat Oncol Biol Phys 2009;73:1270–1275.

85 Bert C, Grozinger SO, Rietzel E: Quantification of interplay effects of scanned particle beams and moving targets. Phys Med Biol 2008;53:2253–2265.

86 Bert C, et al: Dosimetric precision of an ion beam tracking system. Radiat Oncol 2010;5:61.

87 Minohara S, et al: Respiratory gated irradiation system for heavy-ion radiotherapy. Int J Radiat Oncol Biol Phys 2000;47:1097–1103.

88 Jemal A, et al: Global cancer statistics. CA Cancer J Clin 2011;61:69–90.

89 Bujold A, et al: Sequential phase I and II trials of stereotactic body radiotherapy for locally advanced hepatocellular carcinoma. J Clin Oncol 2013;31:1631–1639.

90 Dawson LA, Ten Haken RK: Partial volume tolerance of the liver to radiation. Semin Radiat Oncol 2005;15:279–283.

91 Jung J, et al: Radiation-induced liver disease after stereotactic body radiotherapy for small hepatocellular carcinoma: clinical and dose-volumetric parameters. Radiat Oncol 2013;8:249.

92 Cheng JC, et al: Radiation-induced liver disease after three-dimensional conformal radiotherapy for patients with hepatocellular carcinoma: dosimetric analysis and implication. Int J Radiat Oncol Biol Phys 2002;54:156–162.

93 Dawson LA, et al: Escalated focal liver radiation and concurrent hepatic artery fluorodeoxyuridine for unresectable intrahepatic malignancies. J Clin Oncol 2000;18:2210–2218.

94 Park W, et al: Local radiotherapy for patients with unresectable hepatocellular carcinoma. Int J Radiat Oncol Biol Phys 2005;61:1143–1150.

95 Qi WX, et al: Charged particle therapy versus photon therapy for patients with hepatocellular carcinoma: a systematic review and meta-analysis. Radiother Oncol 2015;114:289–295.

96 Habermehl D, et al: Evaluation of different fiducial markers for image-guided radiotherapy and particle therapy. J Radiat Res 2013;54(suppl 1):i61–i68.

97 Richter D, et al: Four-dimensional patient dose reconstruction for scanned ion beam therapy of moving liver tumors. Int J Radiat Oncol Biol Phys 2014;89:175–181.

98 Hata M, et al: Proton beam therapy for hepatocellular carcinoma with limited treatment options. Cancer 2006;107:591–598.

99 Kato H, et al: Results of the first prospective study of carbon ion radiotherapy for hepatocellular carcinoma with liver cirrhosis. Int J Radiat Oncol Biol Phys 2004;59:1468–1476.

100 Nakayama H, et al: Proton beam therapy for hepatocellular carcinoma: the University of Tsukuba experience. Cancer 2009;115:5499–5506.

101 Bush DA, et al: High-dose proton beam radiotherapy of hepatocellular carcinoma: preliminary results of a phase II trial. Gastroenterology 2004;127(5 suppl 1):S189–S193.

102 Bush DA, et al: The safety and efficacy of high-dose proton beam radiotherapy for hepatocellular carcinoma: a phase 2 prospective trial. Cancer 2011;117:3053–3059.

103 Hong TS, et al: Multi-institutional phase II study of high-dose hypofractionated proton beam therapy in patients with localized, unresectable hepatocellular carcinoma and intrahepatic cholangiocarcinoma. J Clin Oncol 2016;34:460–468.

104 Bush DA, et al: Randomized clinical trial comparing proton beam radiation therapy with transarterial chemoembolization for hepatocellular carcinoma: results of an interim analysis. Int J Radiat Oncol Biol Phys 2016;95:477–482.

105 Sugahara S, et al: Proton-beam therapy for hepatocellular carcinoma associated with portal vein tumor thrombosis. Strahlenther Onkol 2009;185:782–788.

106 Sugahara S, et al: Proton beam therapy for large hepatocellular carcinoma. Int J Radiat Oncol Biol Phys 2010;76:460–466.

107 Kimura K, et al: Clinical results of proton beam therapy for hepatocellular carcinoma over 5 cm. Hepatol Res 2017;47:1368–1374.

108 Fukuda K, et al: Long-term outcomes of proton beam therapy in patients with previously untreated hepatocellular carcinoma. Cancer Sci 2017;108:497–503.

109 Kim DY, et al: Risk-adapted simultaneous integrated boost-proton beam therapy (SIB-PBT) for advanced hepatocellular carcinoma with tumour vascular thrombosis. Radiother Oncol 2017;122:122–129.

110 Oshiro Y, et al: Analysis of repeated proton beam therapy for patients with hepatocellular carcinoma. Radiother Oncol 2017;123:240–245.

111 Combs SE, et al: Phase i study evaluating the treatment of patients with hepatocellular carcinoma (HCC) with carbon ion radiotherapy: the PROMETHEUS-01 trial. BMC Cancer 2011;11:67.

112 Raimondi S, Maisonneuve P, Lowenfels AB: Epidemiology of pancreatic cancer: an overview. Nat Rev Gastroenterol Hepatol 2009;6:699–708.

113 Gillen S, et al: Preoperative/neoadjuvant therapy in pancreatic cancer: a systematic review and meta-analysis of response and resection percentages. PLoS Med 2010;7:e1000267.

114 Habermehl D, et al: Neoadjuvant chemoradiation with gemcitabine for locally advanced pancreatic cancer. Radiat Oncol 2012;7:28.

115 Naumann P, et al: Outcome after neoadjuvant chemoradiation and correlation with nutritional status in patients with locally advanced pancreatic cancer. Strahlenther Onkol 2013;189:745–752.

116 Habermehl D, et al: Chemoradiation in patients with isolated recurrent pancreatic cancer – therapeutical efficacy and probability of re-resection. Radiat Oncol 2013;8:27.

117 Nakamura A, et al: Radiotherapy for patients with isolated local recurrence of primary resected pancreatic cancer: prolonged disease-free interval associated with favorable prognosis. Strahlenther Onkol 2014;190:485–490.

118 Habermehl D, et al: Hypofractionated carbon ion therapy delivered with scanned ion beams for patients with hepatocellular carcinoma – feasibility and clinical response. Radiat Oncol 2013;8:59.

119 Shinoto M, et al: Phase 1 trial of preoperative, short-course carbon-ion radiotherapy for patients with resectable pancreatic cancer. Cancer 2013;119:45–51.

120 Schneider RA, et al: Small bowel toxicity after high dose spot scanning-based proton beam therapy for paraspinal/retroperitoneal neoplasms. Strahlenther Onkol 2013;189:1020–1025.

121 Takatori K, et al: Upper gastrointestinal complications associated with gemcitabine-concurrent proton radiotherapy for inoperable pancreatic cancer. J Gastroenterol 2014;49:1074–1080.

122 Nichols RC Jr, et al: Proton therapy with concomitant capecitabine for pancreatic and ampullary cancers is associated with a low incidence of gastrointestinal toxicity. Acta Oncol 2013;52:498–505.

123 Terashima K, et al: A phase I/II study of gemcitabine-concurrent proton radiotherapy for locally advanced pancreatic cancer without distant metastasis. Radiother Oncol 2012;103:25–31.

124 Hong TS, et al: Phase I study of preoperative short-course chemoradiation with proton beam therapy and capecitabine for resectable pancreatic ductal adenocarcinoma of the head. Int J Radiat Oncol Biol Phys 2011;79:151–157.

125 El Shafie RA, et al: In vitro evaluation of photon and raster-scanned carbon ion radiotherapy in combination with gemcitabine in pancreatic cancer cell lines. J Radiat Res 2013;54(suppl 1):i113–i119.

126 Habermehl D, et al: The relative biological effectiveness for carbon and oxygen ion beams using the raster-scanning technique in hepatocellular carcinoma cell lines. PLoS One 2014; 9:e113591.

127 Oonishi K, et al: Different effects of carbon ion beams and X-rays on clonogenic survival and DNA repair in human pancreatic cancer stem-like cells. Radiother Oncol 2012;105:258–265.

128 Okada T, et al: Carbon ion radiotherapy: clinical experiences at National Institute of Radiological Science (NIRS). J Radiat Res 2010;51:355–364.

129 Shinoto M, et al: Carbon ion radiation therapy with concurrent gemcitabine for patients with locally advanced pancreatic cancer. Int J Radiat Oncol Biol Phys 2016;95:498–504.

130 Mizumoto M, et al: Clinical results of proton-beam therapy for locoregionally advanced esophageal cancer. Strahlenther Onkol 2010;186:482–488.

131 Ishikawa H, et al: Proton beam therapy combined with concurrent chemotherapy for esophageal cancer. Anticancer Res 2015;35:1757–1762.

132 Lin SH, et al: Proton beam therapy and concurrent chemotherapy for esophageal cancer. Int J Radiat Oncol Biol Phys 2012;83:e345–e351.

133 Akutsu Y, et al: A phase I/II clinical trial of preoperative short-course carbon-ion radiotherapy for patients with squamous cell carcinoma of the esophagus. J Surg Oncol 2012;105:750–755.

134 Wong RK, et al: Preoperative or postoperative therapy for stage II or III rectal cancer: an updated practice guideline. Clin Oncol 2010;22:265–271.

135 Yamada S, et al: Current status and perspective of heavy ion beam therapy for patients with pelvic recurrence after primarily resected rectal cancer (in Japanese). Gan To Kagaku Ryoho 2009;36:1263–1266.

136 Yamada S, et al: Carbon-ion radiation therapy for pelvic recurrence of rectal cancer. Int J Radiat Oncol Biol Phys 2016;96:93–101.

137 Vogelius IR, Bentzen SM: Meta-analysis of the alpha/beta ratio for prostate cancer in the presence of an overall time factor: bad news, good news, or no news? Int J Radiat Oncol Biol Phys 2013;85:89–94.

138 Shipley WU, et al: Advanced prostate cancer: the results of a randomized comparative trial of high dose irradiation boosting with conformal protons compared with conventional dose irradiation using photons alone. Int J Radiat Oncol Biol Phys 1995;32:3–12.

139 Slater JD, et al: Proton therapy for prostate cancer: the initial Loma Linda University experience. Int J Radiat Oncol Biol Phys 2004;59:348–352.

140 Slater JD, et al: Conformal proton therapy for prostate carcinoma. Int J Radiat Oncol Biol Phys 1998;42:299–304.

141 Zietman AL, et al: Randomized trial comparing conventional-dose with high-dose conformal radiation therapy in early-stage adenocarcinoma of the prostate: long-term results from Proton Radiation Oncology Group/American College of Radiology 95-09. J Clin Oncol 2010;28:1106–1111.

142 Zietman AL, et al: Comparison of conventional-dose vs high-dose conformal radiation therapy in clinically localized adenocarcinoma of the prostate: a randomized controlled trial. JAMA 2005; 294:1233–1239.

143 Hara I, et al: Experience with conformal proton therapy for early prostate cancer. Am J Clin Oncol 2004;27:323–327.

144 Mendenhall NP, et al: Early outcomes from three prospective trials of image-guided proton therapy for prostate cancer. Int J Radiat Oncol Biol Phys 2012;82:213–221.

145 Talcott JA, et al: Patient-reported long-term outcomes after conventional and high-dose combined proton and photon radiation for early prostate cancer. JAMA 2010;303:1046–1053.

146 Kim YJ, et al: A phase II study of hypofractionated proton therapy for prostate cancer. Acta Oncol 2013;52:477–485

147 Vargas CE, et al: Hypofractionated versus standard fractionated proton-beam therapy for low-risk prostate cancer: interim results of a randomized trial PCG GU 002. Am J Clin Oncol 2018;41:115–120.

148 Yamoah K, Johnstone PA: Proton beam therapy: clinical utility and current status in prostate cancer. Onco Targets Ther 2016;9:5721–5727.

149 Bryant C, et al: Five-year biochemical results, toxicity, and patient-reported quality of life after delivery of dose-escalated image guided proton therapy for prostate cancer. Int J Radiat Oncol Biol Phys 2016;95:422–434.

150 Tsuji H, et al: Hypofractionated radiotherapy with carbon ion beams for prostate cancer. Int J Radiat Oncol Biol Phys 2005;63:1153–1160.

151 Nomiya T, et al: A multi-institutional analysis of prospective studies of carbon ion radiotherapy for prostate cancer: a report from the Japan Carbon Ion Radiation Oncology Study Group (J-CROS). Radiother Oncol 2016;121: 288–293.

152 Okada T, et al: Carbon ion radiotherapy in advanced hypofractionated regimens for prostate cancer: from 20 to 16 fractions. Int J Radiat Oncol Biol Phys 2012;84:968–972.

153 Rucinski A, et al: Ion therapy of prostate cancer: daily rectal dose reduction by application of spacer gel. Radiat Oncol 2015;10:56.

154 Fowler JF: The radiobiology of prostate cancer including new aspects of fractionated radiotherapy. Acta Oncol 2005;44:265–276.

155 Akakura K, et al: Phase I/II clinical trials of carbon ion therapy for prostate cancer. Prostate 2004;58:252–258.

156 Ishikawa H, et al: Carbon ion radiation therapy for prostate cancer: results of a prospective phase II study. Radiother Oncol 2006;81:57–64.

157 Schiller KC, Habl G, Combs SE: Protons, photons, and the prostate – is there emerging evidence in the ongoing discussion on particle therapy for the treatment of prostate cancer? Front Oncol 2016;6:8.

158 Eifel PJ, et al: Pelvic irradiation with concurrent chemotherapy versus pelvic and para-aortic irradiation for high-risk cervical cancer: an update of radiation therapy oncology group trial (RTOG) 90-01. J Clin Oncol 2004;22: 872–880.

159 Kirwan JM, et al: A systematic review of acute and late toxicity of concomitant chemoradiation for cervical cancer. Radiother Oncol 2003;68:217–226.

160 Kagei K, et al: Long-term results of proton beam therapy for carcinoma of the uterine cervix. Int J Radiat Oncol Biol Phys 2003;55:1265–1271.

161 Kato S, et al: Dose escalation study of carbon ion radiotherapy for locally advanced carcinoma of the uterine cervix. Int J Radiat Oncol Biol Phys 2006;65:388–397.

162 Nakano T, et al: The phase I/II clinical study of carbon ion therapy for cancer of the uterine cervix. Cancer J Sci Am 1999;5:362–369.

163 Wakatsuki M, et al: Clinical outcomes of carbon ion radiotherapy for locally advanced adenocarcinoma of the uterine cervix in phase 1/2 clinical trial (protocol 9704). Cancer 2014;120: 1663–1669.

164 Shiba S, et al: Carbon-ion radiotherapy for locally advanced cervical cancer with bladder invasion. J Radiat Res 2016;57:684–690.

165 Buchali A, et al: Impact of the filling status of the bladder and rectum on their integral dose distribution and the movement of the uterus in the treatment planning of gynaecological cancer. Radiother Oncol 1999;52:29–34.

166 Meadows AT, et al: Second neoplasms in survivors of childhood cancer: findings from the Childhood Cancer Survivor Study cohort. J Clin Oncol 2009;27: 2356–2362.

167 Travis LB, et al: Second malignant neoplasms and cardiovascular disease following radiotherapy. J Natl Cancer Inst 2012;104:357–370.

168 Kumar S: Second malignant neoplasms following radiotherapy. Int J Environ Res Public Health 2012;9:4744–4759.

169 Miller KD, et al: Cancer treatment and survivorship statistics, 2016. CA Cancer J Clin 2016;66:271–289.

170 Geenen MM, et al: Medical assessment of adverse health outcomes in long-term survivors of childhood cancer. JAMA 2007;297:2705–2715.

171 Brower JV, et al: Proton therapy and helical tomotherapy result in reduced dose deposition to the pancreas in the setting of cranio-spinal irradiation for medulloblastoma: implications for reduced risk of diabetes mellitus in long-term survivors. Acta Oncol 2015; 54:563–566.

172 Farace P, et al: Supine craniospinal irradiation in pediatric patients by proton pencil beam scanning. Radiother Oncol 2017;123:112–118.

173 Eaton BR, et al: Clinical outcomes among children with standard-risk medulloblastoma treated with proton and photon radiation therapy: a comparison of disease control and overall survival. Int J Radiat Oncol Biol Phys 2016;94:133–138.

174 Merchant TE, et al: Proton versus photon radiotherapy for common pediatric brain tumors: comparison of models of dose characteristics and their relationship to cognitive function. Pediatr Blood Cancer 2008;51:110–117.

175 Johnstone PA, et al: Pediatric CSI: are protons the only ethical approach? Int J Radiat Oncol Biol Phys 2013;87:228–230.

176 Yock TI, et al: Long-term toxic effects of proton radiotherapy for paediatric medulloblastoma: a phase 2 single-arm study. Lancet Oncol 2016;17:287–298.

177 Eaton BR, et al: Endocrine outcomes with proton and photon radiotherapy for standard risk medulloblastoma. Neuro Oncol 2016;18:881–887.

178 Luu QT, et al: Fractionated proton radiation treatment for pediatric craniopharyngioma: preliminary report. Cancer J 2006;12:155–159.

179 MacDonald SM, Yock TI: Proton beam therapy following resection for childhood ependymoma. Childs Nerv Syst 2010;26:285–291.

180 Yock T, et al: Proton radiotherapy for orbital rhabdomyosarcoma: clinical outcome and a dosimetric comparison with photons. Int J Radiat Oncol Biol Phys 2005;63:1161–1168.

181 Laffond C, et al: Quality-of-life, mood and executive functioning after childhood craniopharyngioma treated with surgery and proton beam therapy. Brain Inj 2012;26:270–281.

182 Bishop AJ, et al: Proton beam therapy versus conformal photon radiation therapy for childhood craniopharyngioma: multi-institutional analysis of outcomes, cyst dynamics, and toxicity. Int J Radiat Oncol Biol Phys 2014;90: 354–361.

183 Amsbaugh MJ, et al: Proton therapy for spinal ependymomas: planning, acute toxicities, and preliminary outcomes. Int J Radiat Oncol Biol Phys 2012;83:1419–1424.

184 Mizumoto M, et al: Proton beam therapy for pediatric ependymoma. Pediatr Int 2015;57:567–571.

185 Eaton BR, et al: Use of proton therapy for re-irradiation in pediatric intracranial ependymoma. Radiother Oncol 2015;116:301–308.

186 Macdonald SM, et al: Proton radiotherapy for pediatric central nervous system ependymoma: clinical outcomes for 70 patients. Neuro Oncol 2013;15:1552–1559.

187 Childs SK, et al: Proton radiotherapy for parameningeal rhabdomyosarcoma: clinical outcomes and late effects. Int J Radiat Oncol Biol Phys 2012;82: 635–642.

188 Paulino AC, et al: Long-term effects in children treated with radiotherapy for head and neck rhabdomyosarcoma. Int J Radiat Oncol Biol Phys 2000;48: 1489–1495.

189 Ladra MM, et al: Preliminary results of a phase II trial of proton radiotherapy for pediatric rhabdomyosarcoma. J Clin Oncol 2014;32:3762–3770.

190 Vern-Gross TZ, et al: Patterns of failure in pediatric rhabdomyosarcoma after proton therapy. Int J Radiat Oncol Biol Phys 2016;96:1070–1077.

191 Leiser D, et al: Tumour control and quality of life in children with rhabdomyosarcoma treated with pencil beam scanning proton therapy. Radiother Oncol 2016;120:163–168.

Prof. Stephanie E. Combs
Department of Radiation Oncology, Technische Universität München (TUM)
Klinikum rechts der Isar, Ismaninger Strasse 22
DE–81675 Munich (Germany)
E-Mail stephanie.combs@tum.de

Guckenberger M, Combs SE, Zips D (eds): Advances in Radiotherapy.
Prog Tumor Res. Basel, Karger, 2018, vol 44, pp 105–121 (DOI: 10.1159/000486998)

Advances in Radiation Biology
of Particle Irradiation

Alexander Helm · Walter Tinganelli · Marco Durante

Trento Institute for Fundamental Physics and Applications-National Institute for Nuclear Physics (TIFPA-INFN), University of Trento, Trento, Italy

Abstract

The increasing number of centers providing proton or carbon beam therapy underlines the growing importance of charged particle therapy within the spectrum of cancer radiotherapy. Whereas protons are more widely used around the world, carbon ions, which are known to bear a higher efficacy as compared to protons, are still neglected to some extent, especially due to a lack of clinical data on adverse side effects. Yet, an increasing amount of clinical data indicates the distinguished efficacy of carbon ion therapy. Notwithstanding, the radiobiological mechanisms of particle radiation are not completely understood and lag behind advances in technology, which potentially enable new therapy regimens. However, an increased knowledge is required for their application with maximal benefit and sufficient risk estimation. Differential gene expression, distinct molecular mechanisms and signal pathways in the radiation response, and systemic effects, such as increased immunogenicity, and the possibilities of combined treatments arising from them, are important fields of particle radiobiology in which new discoveries and advances have occurred. These aspects are contemplated with respect to an individualization of radiotherapy; radiation type and treatment regimen might be chosen on the basis of the radiosensitivity of the individual and the cancer type. Here, we provide an update on a few recent findings and advances in particle radiobiology. A comprehensive essay on the basics of particle radiobiology is beyond the scope of this article. The focus is directed on a few subjects currently undergoing intense study and which are of current interest with respect to advances in therapy.

© 2018 S. Karger AG, Basel

Radiotherapy (RT) is widely used among cancer therapies and the growing number of centers around the world providing ion beams for charged particle therapy (CPT) underlines its great appreciation for cancer treatment. The advantage of CPT owes to the peculiar physical features of accelerated particles, mainly the inverted dose-depth profile (Fig. 1a), and the resulting radiobiological effects, which have been elegantly described in several publications so far [1–3]. Today, CPT comprises mainly protons (50 centers

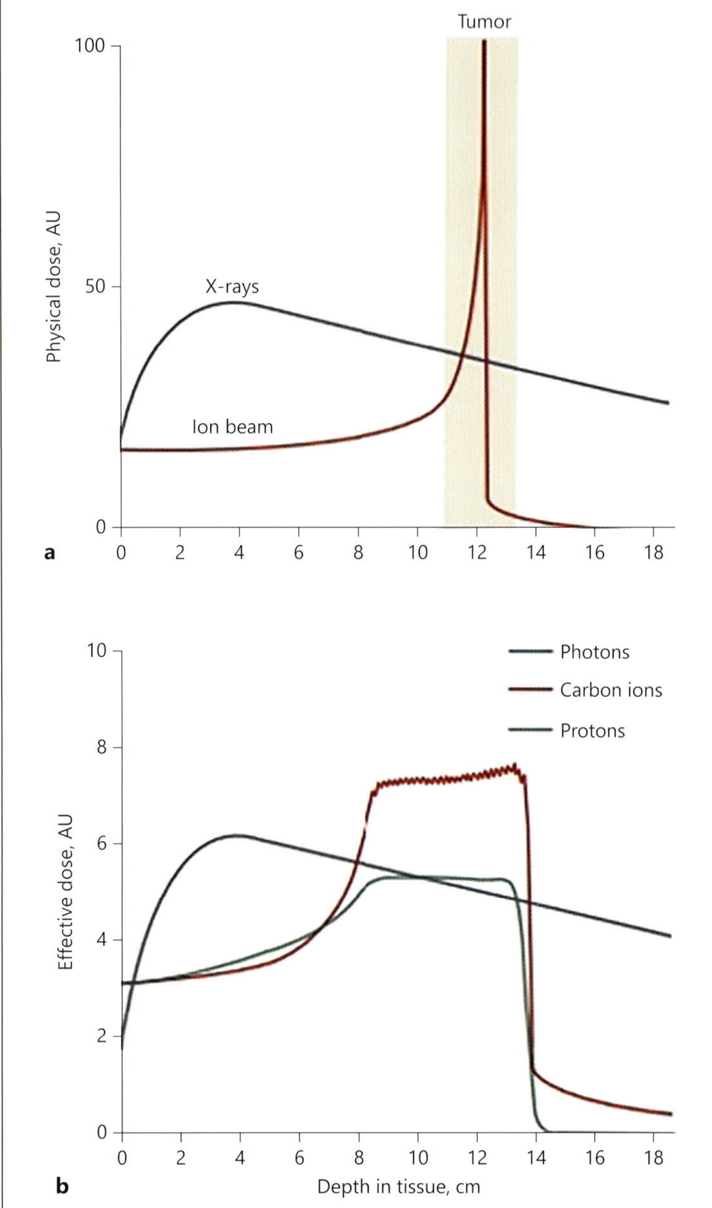

Fig. 1. Schematic dose-depth profile of charged particles. **a** The inverted dose-depth profile of charged particles allows a dose deposition in deep-located tumors. **b** Several Bragg-curves are superimposed to raster a given tumor volume, homogenously distributing the dose. Carbon ions comprise a higher effective dose than protons, but both better spare healthy tissue in the entrance channel. Reprinted with permission from Macmillan Publishers Ltd [2].

worldwide) and to a lesser extent carbon ion beams (6 centers worldwide) [4]. Both particle types offer characteristic advantages and their application is chosen, apart from availability and cost-effectiveness, according to the tumor type, tumor position, and age of the patient. The relative biological effectiveness (RBE; photons are reference radiation) of protons is low (generally considered 1.1). Carbon ions, on the other hand, have an increased RBE owing to the high linear energy transfer (LET), especially in the Bragg peak, whereas the LET in the entrance channel is

Helm · Tinganelli · Durante

rather low. Superimposing Bragg curves results in a spread-out Bragg peak (SOBP), which is used to cover the tumor volume with a homogeneous dose, while being more precise than photon beams and more efficient than protons (Fig. 1b). The fragmentation of a carbon beam is increased as compared to protons, thus resulting in a higher neutron yield. Therefore, pediatric patients are currently treated with protons [2, 5, 6]. Nonetheless, the higher RBE of carbon ions plus the inverted particle dose-depth profile makes them an optimal choice for deep-located radioresistant tumors in adult patients, which are difficult to remove with surgery. Further ion species are currently under investigation for a putative application in therapy, with helium and oxygen being the most promising candidates [7].

The peculiar physical features of charged particles, as opposed to photons, obviously have implications on radiobiological effects. A detailed essay on the basics of the radiobiology of particles is beyond the scope of this work and more details are described elsewhere [1, 2]. Briefly, particle radiation affects the so-called 4 Rs of RT, namely repair, reassortment, reoxygenation, and repopulation, accounting for the high effectiveness of CPT. Due to the clustered DNA damage induced by particles, the repair mechanisms of cells are highly challenged and most cells hit by particles undergo cell death due to misrepair and subsequent chromosomal aberrations. The cells' radiosensitivity depends on the cell cycle, and cells in more resistant phases (late S-phase, G2-phase) might survive a single treatment with photons. In RT, due to the commonly applied temporally separated fractionation, a reassortment (also redistribution) of the cell cycle of targeted tumor cells takes place, thus sensitizing cells by shifting the cell cycle phase. For particle radiation, the cell cycle-dependence of radiosensitivity, however, is mitigated due to the complex DNA damage. Cells in hypoxic compartments of tumors bear a higher radioresistance, and reoxygenation of these cells between the fractions of a therapy regimen normally attenuates such resistance. Particle radiation also more efficiently inactivates hypoxic cells and is hence less dependent on reoxygenation. Finally, tumor cells surviving the treatment may repopulate the tumor site, thus reducing the local tumor control; charged particles, again owing to the higher efficiency in cell inactivation, are believed to have a slightly lower probability for repopulation.

Despite ongoing and increasing research efforts, the biological mechanisms of particle radiobiology are still not completely understood. The classical dogma of cell killing via DNA damage induction has been challenged by recent findings, suggesting an impact of CPT on cell signaling, tumor microenvironment, or systemic effects, for example. The radiation quality influences the cellular response on different levels of complexity. Moreover, new questions arise with advances in technology of beam delivery and image guidance, enabling putative new applications for RT. Here, we provide an overview on recent advances in the knowledge on particle radiobiology and related topics, which are currently the focus of research, as they may provide promising new implications for cancer therapy.

DNA Damage and Repair

The DNA damage induced by particles is based on the dense, localized energy deposition, resulting from the track structure of the respective high-LET particle in contrast to low-LET photons, which deposit the energy sparsely and broadly distributed within a target volume. This basic assumption has hitherto not been questioned, but has rather been refined by studies conducted up to now. Recently, Mirsch et al. [8] elegantly verified the assumptions on the penumbra using a biological 3D model system. The penumbra is the lateral extension of the track's core, which depends on the particle's energy and can increase considerably for highly energetic particles. The assumptions used in radiobiological modelling have mainly been derived from physical measurements in inorganic material and theoretical predictions, which may be considered limited to some extent [9]. The 3D energy deposition was visualized and quantified by staining γH2AX foci, which is a well-established biomarker for DNA damage visualization and biodosimetry [10]. A comparison to the local effect model, a model currently applied in particle cancer therapy for the prediction of the damage induced by heavy ions such as carbon [11], revealed a good conformance of the damage distribution within the penumbra [8]. Their findings also support little damage and high survival probability for exposed tissue located in the penumbra, whereas cells within the track core have a high probability of death. Thus, the cells rather die than undergo transformation, which is one of the evident advantages of CPT. This increased probability of cell death in the track core of the particle is due to the rather complex and clustered DNA damage induced by a high-LET particle as compared with the low LET resulting from the sparsely ionizing photons. An increasing LET elevates the probability for the occurrence of double strand breaks (DSB) in close vicinity. The results are clustered lesions of complex damages consisting of multiple single strand breaks and DSB [12]. The complexity of those lesions subsequently influences the further processing; for example, different recruitment dynamics of early repair proteins following high-LET exposure have been reported [13]. A mammalian cell resorts to mainly 2 DNA repair pathways, namely homologous recombination (HR) and nonhomologous end joining (NHEJ) to counter the induced damage, where NHEJ is considered the predominant pathway since it dominates during the G1-phase and also occurs throughout the whole cell cycle [14]. As for high-LET radiation, the assumed predominance of NHEJ [15] has recently been challenged, as indicated by an increased resection activity in G1-phase cells, suggesting the alternative

NHEJ, also referred to as MMEJ (microhomology-mediated end joining), to be a major yet error-prone (as compared to HR) repair choice when it comes to clustered lesions [16, 17]. Low-LET protons, on the other hand, despite inducing a differential quality of DNA damage as compared to photons, seem to mainly rely on HR for damage repair [18]. Recent experimental evidence [19] underlines the complexity of clustered lesions in heterochromatic regions and the subsequent perturbed repair capacity as a crucial reason for the increased biological effectiveness of high-LET radiation. Using a high-resolution transmission electron microscopy approach with immunogold labelling, Lorat et al. [19–21] elegantly showed the spatially localized concentration of the DSB in complex lesions, since they report not only an increase in the number of clustered lesions but also in cluster size. They showed that the cluster complexity depends on the packing density of DNA along the ion track, leading to complex clusters mainly in condensed heterochromatic regions. The investigation of the successive evolution of these clustered lesions points to a perturbed DNA repair, as indicated by the NHEJ-related repair protein pKu70, leading to a persisting damage in dependence on rather the vicinity than the number of DSB [19, 21]. Notwithstanding, a peculiar process in the repair of those clustered lesions in heterochromatin following high-LET exposure has been shown and was reported to be based on a local chromatin decondensation (i.e., at the damage site), leading to a subsequent relocation of the damage site to the periphery of the affected heterochromatic region. This bending of damage sites around the highly compacted DNA regions is believed to allow for a more efficient recruitment of repair proteins [22]. Incompletely repaired high-LET-induced clustered lesions combined with an impaired cell cycle checkpoint release may contribute to chromosomal aberrations, and thus result in late effects [23]. Nevertheless, high-LET particles yield more complex-type chromosome aberrations, which bear a higher probability for the affected cell of subsequently undergoing cell death [24].

Hypoxia, Resistance, and New Approaches to Overcome It

Most tumors comprise regions with a low oxygen concentration, occurring either in avascular primary tumors and metastases or because of an abnormal tumor vasculature which is spatially disorganized, thus leading to a heterogeneous oxygen concentration throughout the tumor owing to diffusion limitations. A temporal dynamic component in the heterogeneity of the oxygen concentration is further introduced by an unstable blood flow, which leads to fluctuation in the oxygen supply [25]. These dynamics lead to the differentiation between chronic and acute hypoxia for clinical radiobiology and the oxygen deficiency can be either close to 0% or even drop to a complete lack of oxygen [26, 27]. The hypoxia-induced relative radioresistance poses a problem for conventional RT and can be quantified with the oxygen enhancement ratio, i.e. the ratio of iso-effective (mainly cell death) doses in a hypoxic and fully oxygenated condition [28, 29]. However, it has been demonstrated that hypoxia-induced radioresistance can be overcome by high-LET radiation [26, 27]. Therefore, it is assumed that the carbon ion beam is superior to conventional RT when it comes to radioresistant tumors [2, 30], and clinical data demonstrating a similar local tumor control probability (TCP) for oxic and hypoxic cervical cancer after carbon ion therapy seem to be in line with this hypothesis [31]. Furthermore, recent approaches in treatment planning try to redistribute multiple fields in order to enhance the cell killing in the region where the largest hypoxia is located. This is the case for LET-painting [32] and kill-painting [29], the latter being experimentally verified. In order to reach sufficient LET values for treatment planning to overcome hypoxia-related resistance, consideration of using oxygen ions instead of carbon ions has already been implemented in models [32, 33]. Experimental verification is on its way and preliminary data have recently been presented by Scifoni et al. [34]. Hypoxia has also been linked with resistance due to the enhancement of cancer stem cell niches, and high-LET charged particles are considered as a putative strategy targeting cancer stem cells [30].

Normal Tissue Tolerance and Implications for the RBE

A striking advantage of particle therapy is definitely the sparing effect of the normal healthy tissue, reducing the number of entrance fields as compared to RT with photons [2]. This is due to the Bragg peak of charged particles, which allows the delivery of a certain dose to the tumor target volume with a low number of fields, i.e., 1–3, as opposed to photon RT, where intensity-modulated RT may require up to 10 fields [35]. The relevance of sparing with CPT is highlighted when consulting a calculation by Yovino et al. [36], whereupon a single photon RT fraction delivers 0.5 Gy to about 5% of the circulating blood cells. There is convincing evidence for the beneficial sparing, stemming from patients who underwent carbon ion therapy in Japan and Germany, which demonstrates less chromosomal aberrations in the patients' peripheral blood lymphocytes than in patients who were treated with X-rays [37, 38]. Notwithstanding, it should be noted that these findings are not in contradiction with the increased efficiency of heavy ions to induce chromosomal aberrations [24], but are simply owing to the abovementioned sparing effect.

The RBE has ever since been the central parameter for comparison and for to scale data from different radiation qualities. In CPT, the RBE-weighted absorbed dose is nowadays described in Gy (RBE). In proton therapy, a constant RBE value of 1.1 is commonly assumed throughout the SOBP, whereas for carbon ion therapy the RBE varies with the LET along the SOBP [2]. However, the current RBE considerations bear uncertainties. In RT, the normal tissue complication probability (NTCP), as well as the TCP, are calculated based on cell killing effects only. These data stem from studies mainly performed in cell cultures in vitro and exhibit large fluctuations in the RBE-LET relationship when comparing available data sets [39, 40]. When aiming at comparisons between in vitro and in vivo cell survival data, additional confusion is introduced by the nature of the tissues, which are normally the focus of in vivo investigations. These tissues predominantly react early and hence have a high α/β ratio. In contrast, in vitro data are essentiality derived from V79 Chinese hamster cells, typically featuring a low α/β ratio, which subsequently impair comparisons of RBE values that also depend on the α/β ratio [40].

Furthermore, these data are generated by means of clonogenic cell survival, which may well be doubted for its appropriateness as an exclusive representative marker for the side effects of radiation in the normal healthy tissues, which are insufficiently characterized for particles. Simple clonogenic cell survival does not account for radiation impacts on non-targeted effects, such as bystander effects (e.g., cell-cell signaling), genomic instability, immunogenic and inflammatory responses, and changes in the tumor microenvironment (which for example may trigger systemic immunogenic responses, see below) [40–42]. More complex in vivo endpoints, which better reflect the complex situation in a tissue, such as lung fibrosis or spinal cord injury, may be considered more appropriate as factors for calculations of the NTCP in future. Thus, the introduction of new biological parameters for the RBE calculations in the tumor and normal tissue response may subsequently reduce uncertainties. This would not only increase the efficiency of TCP while decreasing the NTCP, but it may also con-

tribute to the individualization of CPT and the identification of patients to benefit from it [40]. Additionally, a better understanding of the normal tissue toxicity would valuably contribute to applications of hypofractionation, as discussed below.

Radiogenomics

There is a general tendency towards an individualization of cancer therapy regimens according to the patient's needs and background. In RT, this is characterized mainly by the effort to exploit radiogenomics, with the ultimate aim of an individual prediction of the patient's radiosensitivity. Information derived from the patient's genome would then allow for an individual adaption, i.e., where possible an increase of the prescribed dose to the tumor (accepting where necessary an increased dose to the normal tissue), optimally leading to an increased TCP while keeping the NTCP level low. A differentiation between the respective radiation response of the tumor and the response of the normal tissue would be ideal with respect to such individualization [43, 44].

Methodically, radiogenomics commonly applies the candidate-gene approach looking for genetic variations within these genes, which are related to the radiation response. The genetic variations that are screened for include, for example, copy number variations, SNP (single nucleotide polymorphism), or epigenetic modifications [45, 46]. A study by Barnett et al. [47], however, contradicts the former findings and questions the association between SNP and individual radiation toxicity. Commonly used candidates include *BRCA1* and *BRCA2*, which are part of the DNA repair response, *TGFB1* as a representative for cytokine production, or *SOD2*, a scavenger of free radicals [48]. Another famous example for a candidate gene is *ATM*, which plays an important role in DSB repair and is homozygously mutated in AT (ataxia-telangectasia) patients, thus inducing an extreme radiosensitivity [49]. Such diseases, however, are rare and not responsible for observed individual differences in radiosensitivity. Nevertheless, it is noteworthy that a fraction of about 3% of the population is heterozygous for *ATM* mutations, while a similar fraction of individuals was found to be hypersensitive in RT trials [35, 50]. Furthermore, studies in mice revealed a radiosensitivity due to *ATM* haploinsufficiency [51, 52]. The *ATM* haploinsufficiency was found to accelerate the cataractogenesis in mice following radiation exposure and high-LET heavy ions were found to have a higher RBE with respect to the acceleration [53], which is one of the few studies available for radiation with a higher LET. Another methodical approach in radiogenomics is represented by microarray analysis of gene expression. Using this approach, a recent study investigated the effects of different radiation qualities on human bronchial epithelial cells, comparing γ-rays to heavy ions (iron and silicon) [54]. Whereas the dose was reported not to be a significant parameter, radiation quality seems to be one, since a differential gene expression pattern was found for all 3 types of radiation. This approach may gain high importance in the future of individual radiation therapy in the decision of whether particle therapy is an appropriate choice.

As a matter of course, radiogenomic studies have also been performed on tumor tissue to predict specific radioresistances. Integrating acquired molecular tumor data with data from TCP in order to define a set of biomarkers for tumor response prediction [44] may represent a milestone towards an individualized RT. On the basis of data from in vitro survival curves of various human tumor cell lines, Amundson et al. [55] described a set of differentially expressed genes applying microarray gene expression profiling, where 18 genes were associated with radioresistance and 22 genes with radiosensitivity. A further study defined a 10-hub network of differentially expressed genes, which may be suitable as biomarkers in 48 cancer cell lines [56]. Such ap-

proaches may finally lead to the indication of which patients predominantly benefit from particle therapy, as they suffer from radioresistant tumors, whose radioresistance is assumed to be mitigated by high-LET particles. A reduced radiosensitivity has been shown in in vitro (tumor cell lines) and ex vivo (organotypic tissue slices from human tumors) studies, where the variance in radiosensitivity due to the genetic background and interindividuality, respectively, was reported to be decreased following an exposure to high-LET particles as compared to photons [57, 58]. Pediatric patients may especially benefit from such diagnostic progress for the definition of an appropriate therapy form, since a potential induction of secondary tumors in radiosensitive individuals particularly matters when exposed at a young age [35]. For those pediatric patients a treatment with proton beam therapy is beneficial as much normal tissue may be spared compared to with photon RT [59].

Late Adverse Effects

Cancer is a disease of aging and the majority of patients treated with RT are at an age where a risk of late radiation-induced morbidity might be a minor concern, as long as the NTCP is kept at acceptable levels with respect to acute effects. However, in the RT treatment of younger cancer patients, where a considerable life span following the treatment is expected, it is a major issue and it is definitely the major concern in the treatment of pediatric patients with charged particles [6]. Whereas the risk of late complications as a result of conventional photon therapy is rather well characterized [60], and was underlined by findings in the atomic bomb survivors for a given range of doses [61], the epidemiological knowledge of results of exposure to high-energy charged particles is rather poor. While on space missions, such as on the International Space Station, astronauts are exposed to particle radiation at a

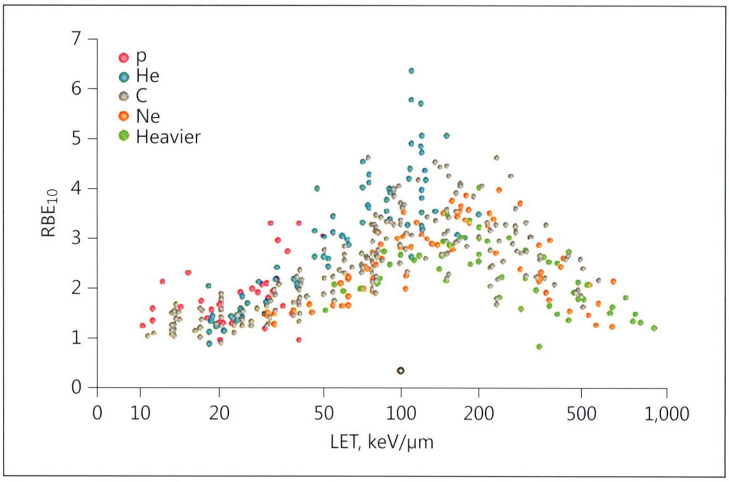

Fig. 2. RBE as a function of the LET. The bell shape is typical for various biological endpoints. The example depicts a 10% clonogenic cell survival as the biological endpoint following exposure to various charged particles at different LET values and are extracted from the PIDE database [39]. Reprinted with permission from Macmillan Publishers Ltd [127].

higher magnitude than on earth, which makes them a relevant cohort for such epidemiological studies. Nevertheless, the doses they are exposed to during their career are relatively low. Consistently, the astronaut cohort did not reveal an increased cancer incidence [62]. A trend towards a reduced risk of second malignancies following proton therapy was found in a cohort of 558 patients, as shown by preliminary study results [63].

Insufficient epidemiological data result in an imprecise risk assessment of CPT. Hence, experimental data, both in vitro and in vivo, are pivotal to contributing to a better understanding of the risk of second malignancies following exposure to particles. As for the in vitro experimental data, a major drawback which needs to be considered is their artificiality, since many experimental systems are based on immortalized or hybrid cell lines. Studies such as in mouse fibroblasts, Syrian hamster embryo fibroblasts, or hybrid CGL1 cells (HeLa X human skin fibroblasts) investigating neoplastic transformation upon exposure to different charged particles commonly result in a typical bell-shaped RBE-LET relationship, as reported for various biological endpoints (Fig. 2) [35]. With an increasing LET, the RBE initially rises until about 100 keV/µm and subsequently decreases, thus accounting for an overkill effect.

Hence, the dose-effect curves for transformation in cell lines is typically linear up to a plateau reached at a certain dose [61, 64]. Comparison of results from animal studies shows that the relationship between dose and the risk of cancer is rather complex and no simple conclusion can be drawn to all species, strains of experimental species, or types of organs. The most valid data stem from mouse studies and show no linear relationship between dose and risk in many cases, as opposed to in vitro data. Generally, the observed heterogeneity in experimental cancer induction in vivo indicates a pivotal role for the individual genetic background [61]. This fact strengthens the great importance for the application of radiogenomics in future RT regimens, as described above. Such heterogeneity is also shown in in vivo data for particle radiation as indicated by different RBE values for the induction of various types of cancer [35]. The RBE of 1 GeV/nucleon iron ions for cancer induction in mice, for example, was reported to be about 1 for murine acute myeloid leukemia (AML) but about 20 for hepatocellular carcinoma (HCC) [65]. Likewise, huge differences in the RBE values of high-energy high-LET ions for the induction of these 2 cancer types were confirmed in a follow-up study and also shown for silicon ions. In the same study, high-energy low-LET protons were found to bear a similar effectiveness to γ-rays, which served as reference radiation [66]. The huge difference in the induction capacity for the 2 tumor types might be explained by the different mechanisms of induction that underlie for liquid (here AML) and solid tumors (here HCC), respectively, as suggested by Weil et al. [66]. AML has been reported as being related to specific chromosomal aberrations, which may represent initiators of carcinogenesis, and it is believed that only a few steps are required for the development of murine AML. Despite the high efficiency for heavy ions in the induction of chromosomal aberrations, many aberrations are lethal and affected cells are subsequently removed by cell death. Thus, the fractions of survivors harboring a specific chromosome aberration needed as an initiator may be similar between photons and heavy ions. HCC, on the other hand, is an epithelial tumor for which a more complex process of carcinogenesis seems to be required based on current knowledge. Radiation-induced cellular alterations and effects on the microenvironment, such as impaired cell signaling or enhanced inflammation, are considered as promotors of carcinogenesis. Heavy ions are known to be rather effective in the induction of inflammation, thus representing more powerful promotors in the development of a solid cancer as compared to photons. Nonetheless, a role of radiation-induced changes of the microenvironment in leukemogenesis cannot be ruled out [35, 66].

The late adverse effects of radiation are not limited to cancer induction. In fact, noncancer diseases are reported to occur following exposure to even low and moderate doses of ionizing radiation as indicated by epidemiological data stemming from the atomic bomb survivors or cohorts of RT patients and occupationally exposed cohorts [67, 68]. Noncancer late adverse effects mainly comprise cataract formation, damage to the central nervous system (CNS), and cardiovascular diseases, but are not restricted to these. Generally, only few epidemiological data are available for particle radiation and the radiobiology behind this is largely unknown.

As for the formation of cataracts, in vivo studies with high-LET particles revealed a high RBE value (up to 50) at relatively low doses [69]. This explains epidemiological evidence from data obtained from astronaut cohorts showing that space radiation (where particle radiation is the predominant component) leads to the opacification of the lens [70]. High-LET particles, already at low doses, may result not only in an increased incidence of cataracts, but also in a reduced latency, and the age at exposure seems to be important [71]. The existence of a threshold cannot be excluded but the actual dose-response relationship remains to be elucidated [72].

Adverse effects on the CNS after cranial RT, such as necrosis and leukoencephalopathy, with the latter being related to cognitive deficits, have been known for decades and were reported not only following photon but also after proton therapy [73–76]. For heavy ions, cognitive deficits in animals have been described after relatively low doses [77, 78]. The various effects on cognitive efficiency and behavior in rats after exposure to different ions were reviewed by Rabin et al. [79]. There is experimental evidence that radiation compromises the structural complexity and synaptic integrity of neurons. A reduction in dendritic complexity and dendritic spine density have been reported both for photons and protons [80, 81]. These alterations seem to also occur already after exposure to low doses of heavy ions [82, 83] and coincided with an increased expression of the protein PSD-95 [83], which operates centrally in the organization of the synaptic function [84]. The abovementioned changes in the neuronal structure were found to be correlated to cognitive deficits and data indicate a certain susceptibility of the CNS to heavy ion exposure. The complex spatial structure of the neurons in the CNS together with the track structure of the high LET particles and the resulting cross-section might account for this efficiency [83]. Although the biological mechanisms in the pathogenesis remain to be elucidated, there are experimental hints for an involvement of oxidative stress and mitochondrial dysfunction after proton exposure [81, 85] as well as a neuroinflammatory response after low doses of iron ions and/or protons [86, 87]. However, it has so far been difficult to draw any conclusions for a putative RBE estimation, since the effects are rather complex and the dose-response relation is still unclear [35, 79]. For high doses of carbon ions instead, where the rat spinal cord and a subsequent paresis were used as a model system, an increase of the RBE with the LET has been reported [88]. It should be noted, though, that another possible mechanism for the induction of adverse late effects in the CNS and cognitive dysfunction is believed to be related with vascular damage induced by RT [89].

It is well known that an exposure of the heart during RT may result in cardiovascular disease, typically evolving after a long latency. This has been shown for high doses up to 30 Gy [90], but epidemiological data from breast cancer patients suggest that cardiovascular disease may also occur for doses to the heart below 2 Gy [91]. A significant increased risk has been suggested even for doses around 0.5 Gy, and the majority of data point to a linear no-threshold dose response; however, a threshold cannot be ruled out based on current knowledge [92]. This underlines the importance to spare the heart and main vessels in its vicinity during RT. Breast cancer therapy using photons, for example, may lead to a significant radiation exposure of the heart [91], but particle therapy, namely carbon [93] and more importantly protons [94], represents a powerful tool for efficiently reducing normal tissue toxicity to the heart. Indeed, breast cancer treatment is increasingly focusing on proton therapy [95, 96]. Epidemiologic and experimental data on the adverse cardiac effects of high-LET particles are virtually unavailable, yet it is of certain interest since carbon ions are discussed as a promising future application for catheter-free ablation of atrial fibrillation [97–99], where adjacent cardiac tissue not in the target volume will be exposed to a certain dose.

Several types of cardiac disease have been reported after RT [92], and ischemic heart disease represents an abundant type among those. Ischemic heart disease is characterized by a limitation in the blood flow, thus causing severe adverse effects in the heart. The origin of the blood flow limitation is atherosclerosis, i.e., the formation of atherosclerotic plaques in the arteries. Initial endothelial alteration and inflammation likely play a crucial role in atherogenesis [100, 101]; in fact, according to available data, endothelial radiation damage and a subsequent proinflammatory response likely account for radiation-induced cardiovascular disease [102–104]. Furthermore, experimental in vivo studies demonstrate an accelerated atherosclerotic plaque formation, both after exposure to photons [105] and iron ions in an ApoE$^{-/-}$ mouse model [106]. Adverse effects, however, may not be restricted to the endothelium. The effects of ionizing radiation on cardiomyocytes, especially on the electrophysiology, for example, have barely been studied. There is evidence that abnormalities in conductivity may occur after RT [107], but the mechanism remains to be elucidated. In a recent work, Bakshi et al. [108] demonstrated that in mouse hearts the expression patterns of proteins related to cytoskeletal structure, cell-to-cell signaling, and cellular interaction, which play a major role in the conductivity of cardiomyocytes, were mostly perturbed following the exposure of mice to doses of 0.5 Gy. Interestingly, high doses of carbon ions were reported to partly restore the damage induced by myocardial infarction by upregulation of expression and structural remodeling of the gap junction-forming protein connexin 43 in rabbit hearts, subsequently leading to an increased electrophysiological conductivity [109, 110]. A study by Ghobadi et al. [111] further highlights the importance of sparing the heart from radiation during RT as they report radiation-induced damage in the myocardium and the cardiac vasculature in rats after exposure to proton beams, which became manifest in heart malfunction and perivascular fibrosis. The authors furthermore demonstrated a mutual synergistic damage effect in the induction of heart malfunction, inflammation, and fibrosis when irradiating both the heart and lungs, thus underlining once more the significance of reducing normal tissue toxicity.

Generally, fibrosis, for example featuring reduced elasticity, a diffusion limit of small molecules across membranes, and organ stricture, is a well-known consequence of radiation and a limiting factor to therapy [112]. A reduced integral dose to the normal tissue during RT, as provided by particle therapy, is thus obviously beneficial, but a putative different mechanism of action in the normal tissue requires further investigation. An in vitro study by Fournier et al. [113] reported no indications for higher RBE values of carbon ions in therapy-relevant energies with respect to fibrosis. However, this finding has recently been challenged by an in vivo study using a mouse model, where the RBE value of carbon ions obtained for fibrosis was found to be increased to about 1.5 [114].

Systemic Immune Response and Combined Treatments

Combining CPT and chemotherapy may result in powerful anticancer strategies. A combination between CPT and temozolomide, for example, is currently being tested in several clinical trials for glioblastoma therapy and seems to be promising [115]. Such a combinational approach is considered highly promising as well for the treatment of pancreatic cancer [116]. Most research, however, is currently underway for another form of combined CPT treatment and is related to a systemic immunogenic response. RT has traditionally been regarded as a local treatment to remove tumors or at least to control their growth when applied as palliative therapy. This traditional view, however, is now questioned due to the immunogenic effects, which ionizing radiation bears and which may lead to a systemic response in the RT patient's body. This systemic effect has already occasionally been reported following RT [117] and is characterized by the shrinkage of distal metastases which are located outside the radiation field. Therefore, the effect is referred to as the abscopal effect (Latin ab – away from, Greek scopus – target) and is believed to be due to an activation of the host's immune system. It is now accepted that radiation per se has a certain potential of immunogenicity. The increased immunogenicity stems from several molecular processes that are influenced by radiation, among them being the translocation of calreticulin to the cell membrane, the release of DAMPs (damage-associated molecular patterns), such as the protein HMGB1 and ATP in the tumor stroma. Additionally, radiation modifies the antigen presentation on the cell surface, such as an increased presentation of MHC-I molecules, which present tumor antigens. After the priming of cytotoxic lymphocytes by mature dendritic cells in the lymph nodes and a subsequent clonal expansion, they can travel to the tumor and the metastatic sites, where they induce cell elimination. Additionally, via upregulation of various further molecules, radiation leads to increased tumor infiltration and the facilitation of tumor cell elimination by natural killer cells [118, 119]. This may lead to a reversion of the so-called immunoediting of cancers, a 3-phased process by which cancer cells escape from immunoselection pressure and circumvent elimination by the immune system, both in the primary tumor and the metastases [120].

Nevertheless, ionizing radiation is Janus-faced since it is both immunogenic and triggers immune-suppressive signaling at the same time. Suppressive signaling is caused by the activation of TGFβ, STAT3, BCL-XL, or VEGF, for example, triggering processes which result in the suppression of dendritic cell activation by myeloid-derived suppressor cells and regulatory T cells [118, 119]. The complex immunogenic and immune-suppressive signaling involves many pathways and molecules and was reviewed by Durante et al. [118].

It has been hypothesized that particle radiation may possess a higher potential of immunogenicity than photons, which is believed to be due to the clustered-type DNA damage leading to different DNA damage responses. Likewise, it is assumed that high doses of particle radiation (as they might be applied in stereotactic body radiation therapy [SBRT] or extreme hypofractionation, for example) are even more beneficial with respect to immunogenicity owing to the distinct DNA damage response. A dose dependency of the radiation-induced immunogenicity has recently been demonstrated by Golden et al. [121]. Indeed, the particular damage type induced by heavy ions effectively kills tumor cells, thus potentially enhancing the presentation of tumor antigens and immunogenic processes [122–124]. Data from a recent in vitro study suggest that protons induce such immunogenic effects [125]. There is also evidence from preclinical results which underline the hypothesis of an increased effectiveness in the induction of immunogenicity by carbon ions, as reviewed by Shimokawa et al. [126]. Furthermore, an abscopal metastatic regression has also been found in a patient after carbon ion therapy at NIRS in Japan; the case was reported by Dr. Shigeru Yamada and was described by Durante et al. [118].

Due to the reduced integral doses delivered with CPT, more lymphocytes and other immune cells will certainly be spared (see above) and thus be available for an immune response. In addition, when applied in a few fractions or a single fraction only, the probability of impairing immune cells is further reduced [118, 127]. These features indicate that hypofractionation/SBRT (see below) are promising RT regimens to trigger immunogenicity for the distal treatment of metastases.

In order to successfully exploit the abovementioned features for therapy against metastatic cancer where the primary tumor may be targeted with CPT, it is essential to enhance the stimulation of the immune response and/or to counter immune-suppressive signaling by combination with immunotherapy. There are various immunotherapeutic medicaments available for cancer therapy, some of which are currently being investigated in combination with RT in clinical trials [128], after several clinical cases were reported where such a combination was successful [129]. In summary, a combination of CPT with immunotherapeutic adjuvants offers a promising therapy regimen.

Hypofractionation and SBRT

Remarkable improvements in the technology of beam delivery and imaging, which allow for a better tumor delineation, have led to a tendency to hypofractionation, i.e., a reduced number of but increased dose per fraction. Techniques such as X-ray SBRT may eventually lead to oligofractionation, which is the application of 1–3 fractions with rather high doses of about 25–30 Gy [35]. The biological effects of such high doses are not fully understood, but processes beyond primary tumor cell killing due to DNA damage likely account for the encouraging results in TCP that have been reported so far. A crucial target for high doses of ionizing radiation in the tumor seems to be the vasculature, which is structurally and functionally abnormal and distinct from normal vessels in the tissue [123]. Experimental results show that the tumor vasculature is more vulnerable to radiation than the normal vasculature. Microvascular damage, via a distinct mechanism of cell death, i.e., the ceramide pathway, is pivotal in the high-dose radiation response of a tumor and eventually leads to indirect cell death caused by the deterioration of the intratumor environment [123, 130, 131]. The ceramide pathway, which is orchestrated by acid sphingomyelinase and where ceramide acts as a second messenger to induce apoptosis, seems to be a main pathway especially in the response to high doses [132]. In addition, such indirect cell death seems to be enhanced by an increased immunogenic cell death after SBRT, leading to further cell death in the primary tumor as well as metastases (see above) [122, 123].

The advantage of CPT with respect to sparing healthy surrounding tissue and a high TCP (see above) aligns perfectly with the aims of hypofractionation and SBRT (also referred to as stereotactic ablative RT, or SABR), respectively. It is worth noting that with respect to the distinct mechanisms of additional (indirect) cell death, as mentioned above, high-LET particles are perhaps the most powerful. They are supposed to be more immunogenic than low-LET radiation (see above) and have been found to be efficient in cell killing of endothelial cells in vitro [133] and damaging of vessel-like structures in a 3D in vitro model [134]. High-LET particles have additionally been shown to efficiently induce the ceramide pathway in tumor cells [135, 136]. In fact, the results of studies in which protons and predominantly carbon ions have been applied in SBRT are highly promising with respect to TCP and side effects, and have been reviewed elsewhere [35, 137].

Conclusion

Much research activity in the field of particle radiobiology is ongoing, with the aim of improving therapy regimens or to set up new ones. However, much more research will be needed to better understand and subsequently exploit the vast possibilities offered by CTP. A comprehensive review of all the research currently underway or needed is beyond the scope of this article. However, we have highlighted topics that are currently in the focus of research. The topics comprise differential gene expression, distinct molecular mechanisms, and signal pathways in the response to particle radiation, systemic effects such as an increased immunogenicity, and the resulting possibilities of combined treatments. An increased application of CPT is foreseeable in the future and can perfectly match with the tendency towards an individualization of RT.

References

1 Fokas E, Kraft G, An H, Engenhart-Cabillic R: Ion beam radiobiology and cancer: time to update ourselves. Biochim Biophys Acta 2009;1796:216–229.

2 Durante M, Loeffler JS: Charged particles in radiation oncology. Nat Rev Clin Oncol 2010;7:37–43.

3 Schardt D, Elsässer T, Schulz-Ertner D: Heavy-ion tumor therapy: physical and radiobiological benefits. Rev Mod Phys 2010;82:383–425.

4 Kamada T, Tsujii H, Blakely EA, Debus J, De Neve W, Durante M, et al: Carbon ion radiotherapy in Japan: an assessment of 20 years of clinical experience. Lancet Oncol 2015;16:e93–e100.

5 Weber U, Kraft G: Comparison of carbon ions versus protons. Cancer J 2009; 15:325–32.

6 Newhauser WD, Durante M: Assessing the risk of second malignancies after modern radiotherapy. Nat Rev Cancer 2011;11:438–48.

7 Tommasino F, Scifoni E, Durante M: New ions for therapy. Int J Part Ther 2015;2:428–438.

8 Mirsch J, Tommasino F, Frohns A, Conrad S, Durante M, Scholz M, et al: Direct measurement of the 3-dimensional DNA lesion distribution induced by energetic charged particles in a mouse model tissue. Proc Natl Acad Sci USA 2015;112:12396–12401.

9 Emfietzoglou D, Moscovitch M: Secondary electron spectra for fast proton impact on gaseous and liquid water. Nucl Instrum Methods Phys Res Sect B 2003; 209:239–245.

10 Barnard S, Ainsbury EA, Al-Hafidh J, Hadjidekova V, Hristova R, Lindholm C, et al: The first gamma-H2AX biodosimetry intercomparison exercise of the developing European biodosimetry network RENEB. Radiat Prot Dosimetry 2015;164:265–270.

11 Tommasino F, Friedrich T, Scholz U, Taucher-Scholz G, Durante M, Scholz M: Application of the local effect model to predict DNA double-strand break rejoining after photon and high-LET irradiation. Radiat Prot Dosimetry 2015; 166:66–70.

12 Hada M, Georgakilas AG: Formation of clustered DNA damage after high-LET irradiation: a review. J Radiat Res 2008; 49:203–210.

13 Tobias F, Löb D, Lengert N, Durante M, Drossel B, Taucher-Scholz G, et al: Spatiotemporal dynamics of early DNA damage response proteins on complex DNA lesions. PLoS One 2013;8:e57953.

14 Branzei D, Foiani M: Regulation of DNA repair throughout the cell cycle. Nat Rev Mol Cell Biol 2008;9:297–308.

15 Takahashi A, Kubo M, Ma H, Nakagawa A, Yoshida Y, Isono M, et al: Nonhomologous end-joining repair plays a more important role than homologous recombination repair in defining radiosensitivity after exposure to high-LET radiation. Radiat Res 2014;182:338–344.

16 Durante M, Bedford JS, Chen DJ, Conrad S, Cornforth MN, Natarajan AT, et al: From DNA damage to chromosome aberrations: joining the break. Mutat Res 2013;756:5–13.

17 Averbeck NB, Ringel O, Herrlitz M, Jakob B, Durante M, Taucher-Scholz G: DNA end resection is needed for the repair of complex lesions in G1-phase human cells. Cell Cycle 2014;13:2509–2516.

18 Grosse N, Fontana AO, Hug EB, Lomax A, Coray A, Augsburger M, et al: Deficiency in homologous recombination renders mammalian cells more sensitive to proton versus photon irradiation. Int J Radiat Oncol Biol Phys 2014;88:175–181.

19 Lorat Y, Timm S, Jakob B, Taucher-Scholz G, Rübe CE: Clustered double-strand breaks in heterochromatin perturb DNA repair after high linear energy transfer irradiation. Radiother Oncol 2016;121:154–161.

20 Lorat Y, Schanz S, Schuler N, Wennemuth G, Rübe C, Rübe CE: Beyond repair foci: DNA double-strand break repair in euchromatic and heterochromatic compartments analyzed by transmission electron microscopy. PLoS One 2012;7:e38165.

21 Lorat Y, Brunner CU, Schanz S, Jakob B, Taucher-Scholz G, Rübe CE: Nanoscale analysis of clustered DNA damage after high-LET irradiation by quantitative electron microscopy – the heavy burden to repair. DNA Repair 2015;28:93–106.

22 Jakob B, Splinter J, Conrad S, Voss KO, Zink D, Durante M, et al: DNA double-strand breaks in heterochromatin elicit fast repair protein recruitment, histone H2AX phosphorylation and relocation to euchromatin. Nucleic Acids Res 2011; 39:6489–6499.

23 Asaithamby A, Hu B, Chen DJ: Unrepaired clustered DNA lesions induce chromosome breakage in human cells. Proc Natl Acad Sci USA 2011;108:8293–8298.

24 Ritter S, Durante M: Heavy-ion induced chromosomal aberrations: a review. Mutat Res 2010;701:38–46.

25 Wilson WR, Hay MP: Targeting hypoxia in cancer therapy. Natur Rev Cancer 2011;11:393–410.

26 Ma NY, Tinganelli W, Maier A, Durante M, Kraft-Weyrather W: Influence of chronic hypoxia and radiation quality on cell survival. J Radiat Res 2013;54: 13–22.

27 Tinganelli W, Ma N-Y, von Neubeck C, Maier A, Schicker C, Kraft-Weyrather W, et al: Influence of chronic hypoxia and radiation quality on cell survival. J Radiat Res 2013;54:23–30.

28 McKeown SR: Defining normoxia, physoxia and hypoxia in tumours – Implications for treatment response. Br J Radiol 2014;87:20130676.

29 Tinganelli W, Durante M, Hirayama R, Krämer M, Maier A, Kraft-Weyrather W, et al: Kill-painting of hypoxic tumours in charged particle therapy. Sci Rep 2015;5:17016.

30 Pignalosa D, Durante M: Overcoming resistance of cancer stem cells. Lancet Oncol 2012;13:e187–e188.

31 Nakano T, Suzuki Y, Ohno T, Kato S, Suzuki M, Morita S, et al: Carbon beam therapy overcomes the radiation resistance of uterine cervical cancer originating from hypoxia. Clin Cancer Res 2006; 12:2185–2190.

32 Bassler N, Toftegaard J, Lühr A, Sørensen BS, Scifoni E, Krämer M, et al: LET-painting increases tumour control probability in hypoxic tumours. Acta Oncol 2014;53:25–32.

33 Scifoni E, Tinganelli W, Weyrather WK, Durante M, Maier A, Krämer M: Including oxygen enhancement ratio in ion beam treatment planning: model implementation and experimental verification. Phys Med Biol 2013;58:3871–3895.

34 Scifoni E, Sokol O, Grün R, Friedrich T, Scholz M, Tinganelli W, et al: Helium and Oxygen beam models in TRiP98: implementation, treatment planning tests and experimental verification. Radiother Oncol 2016;118:S96.

35 Durante M: New challenges in high-energy particle radiobiology. Br J Radiol 2014;87.

36 Yovino S, Kleinberg L, Grossman SA, Narayanan M, Ford E: The etiology of treatment-related lymphopenia in patients with malignant gliomas: modeling radiation dose to circulating lymphocytes explains clinical observations and suggests methods of modifying the impact of radiation on immune cells. Cancer Invest 2013;31:140–144.

37 Durante M, Yamada S, Ando K, Furusawa Y, Kawata T, Majima H, et al: X-rays vs. carbon-ion tumor therapy: cytogenetic damage in lymphocytes. Int J Radiat Oncol Biol Phys 2000;47:793–798.

38 Hartel C, Nikoghosyan A, Durante M, Sommer S, Nasonova E, Fournier C, et al: Chromosomal aberrations in peripheral blood lymphocytes of prostate cancer patients treated with IMRT and carbon ions. Radiother Oncol 2010;95: 73–78.

39 Friedrich T, Scholz U, Elsässer T, Durante M, Scholz M: Systematic analysis of RBE and related quantities using a database of cell survival experiments with ion beam irradiation. J Radiat Res 2013;54:494–514.

40 Tommasino F, Durante M: Proton radiobiology. Cancers (Basel) 2015;7:353–381.

41 Prise KM, O'Sullivan JM: Radiation-induced bystander signalling in cancer therapy. Nat Rev Cancer 2009;9:351–360.

42 Morgan WF, Sowa MB: Non-targeted effects induced by ionizing radiation: mechanisms and potential impact on radiation induced health effects. Cancer Lett 2015;356:17–21.

43 Bentzen SM: Preventing or reducing late side effects of radiation therapy: radiobiology meets molecular pathology. Nat Rev Cancer 2006;6:702–713.

44 Das AK, Bell MH, Nirodi CS, Story MD, Minna JD: Radiogenomics predicting tumor responses to radiotherapy in lung cancer. Semin Radiat Oncol 2010;20: 149–155.

45 Katsanis SH, Katsanis N: Molecular genetic testing and the future of clinical genomics. Nat Rev Genet 2013;14:415–426.

46 The Wellcome Trust Case Control Consortium: Genome-wide association study of CNVs in 16,000 cases of eight common diseases and 3,000 shared controls. Nature 2010;464:713–720.

47 Barnett GC, Coles CE, Elliott RM, Baynes C, Luccarini C, Conroy D, et al: Independent validation of genes and polymorphisms reported to be associ ated with radiation toxicity: a prospective analysis study. Lancet Oncol 2012; 13:65–77.

48 Alsner J, Andreassen CN, Overgaard J: Genetic markers for prediction of normal tissue toxicity after radiotherapy. Semin Radiat Oncol 2008;18:126–135.

49 Pollard JM, Gatti RA: Clinical radiation sensitivity with DNA repair disorders: an overview. Int J Radiat Oncol Biol Phys 2009;74:1323–1331.

50 Swift M, Morrell D, Massey RB, Chase CL: Incidence of cancer in 161 families affected by ataxia-telangiectasia. N Engl J Med 1991;325:1831–1836.

51 Barlow C, Eckhaus MA, Schäffer AA, Wynshaw-Boris A: *Atm* haploinsufficiency results in increased sensitivity to sublethal doses of ionizing radiation in mice. Nat Genet 1999;21:359–360.

52 Worgul B V, Smilenov L, Brenner DJ, Junk A, Zhou W, Hall EJ: *Atm* heterozygous mice are more sensitive to radiation-induced cataracts than are their wild-type counterparts. Proc Natl Acad Sci USA 2002;99:9836–9839.

53 Hall EJ, Worgul BV, Smilenov L, Elliston CD, Brenner DJ: The relative biological effectiveness of densely ionizing heavy-ion radiation for inducing ocular cataracts in wild type versus mice heterozygous for the ATM gene. Radiat Environ Biophys 2006;45:99–104.

54 Ding L-H, Park S, Peyton M, Girard L, Xie Y, Minna JD, et al: Distinct transcriptome profiles identified in normal human bronchial epithelial cells after exposure to γ-rays and different elemental particles of high Z and energy. BMC Genomics 2013;14:372.

55 Amundson SA, Do KT, Vinikoor LC, Lee RA, Koch-Paiz CA, Ahn J, et al: Integrating global gene expression and radiation survival parameters across the 60 cell lines of the National Cancer Institute Anticancer Drug Screen. Cancer Res 2008;68:415–424.

56 Eschrich S, Zhang H, Zhao H, Boulware D, Lee J, Bloom G, et al: Systems biology modeling of the radiation sensitivity network: a biomarker discovery platform. Int J Radiat Oncol Biol Phys 2009; 75:497–505.

57 Weyrather WK, Ritter S, Scholz M, Kraft G: RBE for carbon track-segment irradiation in cell lines of differing repair capacity. Int J Radiat Biol 1999,75.1357 1364.

58 Merz F, Gaunitz F, Dehghani F, Renner C, Meixensberger J, Gutenberg A, et al: Organotypic slice cultures of human glioblastoma reveal different susceptibilities to treatments. Neuro Oncol 2013; 15:670–681.

59 Merchant TE: Clinical controversies: proton therapy for pediatric tumors. Semin Radiat Oncol 2013;23:97–108.

60 Newhauser WD, de Gonzalez AB, Schulte R, Lee C: A review of radiotherapy-induced late effects research after advanced technology treatments. Front Oncol 2016;6:13.

61 Suit H, Goldberg S, Niemierko A, Ancukiewicz M, Hall E, Goitein M, et al: Secondary carcinogenesis in patients treated with radiation: a review of data on radiation-induced cancers in human, non-human primate, canine and rodent subjects. Radiat Res 2007;167:12–42.

62 Durante M, Cucinotta FA: Heavy ion carcinogenesis and human space exploration. Nat Rev Cancer 2008;8:465–72.

63 Chung CS, Yock TI, Nelson K, Xu Y, Keating NL, Tarbell NJ: Incidence of second malignancies among patients treated with proton versus photon radiation. Int J Radiat Oncol Biol Phys 2013;87:46–52.

64 Bettega D, Calzolari P, Hessel P, Stucchi CG, Weyrather WK: Neoplastic transformation induced by carbon ions. Int J Radiat Oncol Biol Phys 2009;73:861–868.

65 Weil MM, Bedford JS, Bielefeldt-Ohmann H, Ray FA, Genik PC, Ehrhart EJ, et al: Incidence of acute myeloid leukemia and hepatocellular carcinoma in mice irradiated with 1 GeV/nucleon ^{56}Fe ions. Radiat Res 2009;172:213–219.

66 Weil MM, Ray FA, Genik PC, Yu Y, McCarthy M, Fallgren CM, et al: Effects of 28Si ions, ^{56}Fe ions, and protons on the induction of murine acute myeloid leukemia and hepatocellular carcinoma. PLoS One 2014;9:e104819.

67 Little MP, Azizova T V, Bazyka D: Systematic review and meta-analysis of circulatory disease from exposure to low-level ionizing radiation and estimates of potential population mortality risks. Environ Health Perspect 2012;120: 1503–1511.

68 Little MP: A review of non-cancer effects, especially circulatory and ocular diseases. Radiat Environ Biophys 2013; 52.135 449.

69 Brenner DJ, Medvedovsky C, Huang Y, Merriam GJ, Worgul BV: Accelerated heavy particles and the lens. VI. RBE studies at low doses. Radiat Res 1991; 128:73–81.

70 Chylack LTJ, Feiveson AH, Peterson LE, Tung WH, Wear ML, Marak LJ, et al: NASCA report 2: longitudinal study of relationship of exposure to space radiation and risk of lens opacity. Radiat Res 2012;178:25–32.

71 Dynlacht JR, Valluri S, Garrett J, Mendonca MS, Lopez JT, Caperell-Grant A, et al: Age and hormonal status as determinants of cataractogenesis induced by ionizing radiation. I. Densely ionizing (high-LET) radiation. Radiat Res 2011; 175:37–43.

72 Blakely EA, Kleiman NJ, Neriishi K, Chodick G, Chylack LT, Cucinotta FA, et al: Radiation cataractogenesis: epidemiology and biology. Radiat Res 2010;173: 709–717.

73 Soussain C, Ricard D, Fike JR, Mazeron JJ, Psimaras D, Delattre JY: CNS complications of radiotherapy and chemotherapy. Lancet 2009;374:1639–1651.

74 Butler JM, Rapp SR, Shaw EG: Managing the cognitive effects of brain tumor radiation therapy. Curr Treat Options Oncol 2006;7:517–523.

75 Meyers CA: Neurocognitive dysfunction in cancer patients. Oncology 2000;14: 75–79.

76 Gridley DS, Grover RS, Loredo LN, Wroe AJ, Slater JD: Proton-beam therapy for tumors of the CNS. Expert Rev Neurother 2010;10:3129–3330.

77 Britten RA, Davis LK, Jewell JS, Miller VD, Hadley MM, Sanford LD, et al: Exposure to mission relevant doses of 1 GeV/nucleon ^{56}Fe particles leads to impairment of attentional set-shifting performance in socially mature rats. Radiat Res 2014;182:292–298.

78 Tseng BP, Giedzinski E, Izadi A, Suarez T, Lan ML, Tran KK, et al: Functional consequences of radiation-induced oxidative stress in cultured neural stem cells and the brain exposed to charged particle irradiation. Antioxid Redox Signal 2014;20:1410–1422.

79 Rabin BM, Shukitt-Hale B, Joseph JA, Carrihill-Knoll KL, Carey AN, Cheng V: Relative effectiveness of different particles and energies in disrupting behavioral performance. Radiat Environ Biophys 2007;46:173–177.

80 Parihar VK, Limoli CL: Cranial irradiation compromises neuronal architecture in the hippocampus. Proc Natl Acad Sci USA 2013;110:12822–12827.

81 Parihar VK, Pasha J, Tran KK, Craver BM, Acharya MM, Limoli CL: Persistent changes in neuronal structure and synaptic plasticity caused by proton irradiation. Brain Struct Funct 2014;220:1161–1171.

82 Allen R, Raber J, Chakraborti A, Fike JR: Fe irradiation alters spine density and dendritic complexity in the mouse hippocampus. Radiat Res 2015;184:586–594.

83 Parihar VK, Allen B, Tran KK, Macaraeg TG, Chu EM, Kwok SF, et al: What happens to your brain on the way to Mars. Sci Adv 2015;1:e1400256.

84 Charych EI, Akum BF, Goldberg JS, Jörnsten RJ, Rongo C, Zheng JQ, et al: Activity-independent regulation of dendrite patterning by postsynaptic density protein PSD-95. J Neurosci 2006;26:10164–10176.

85 Parihar VK, Allen BD, Tran KK, Chmielewski NN, Craver BM, Martirosian V, et al: Targeted overexpression of mitochondrial catalase prevents radiation-induced cognitive dysfunction. Antioxid Redox Signal 2015;22:78–91.

86 Rola R, Fishman K, Baure J, Rosi S, Lamborn KR, Obenaus A, et al: Hippocampal neurogenesis and neuroinflammation after cranial irradiation with ⁵⁶Fe particles. Radiat Res 2008;169:626–632.

87 Raber J, Allen AR, Sharma S, Allen B, Rosi S, Olsen RHJ, et al: Effects of proton and combined proton and ⁵⁶Fe radiation on the hippocampus. Radiat Res 2016;185:20–30.

88 Saager M, Glowa C, Peschke P, Brons S, Grün R, Scholz M, et al: Split dose carbon ion irradiation of the rat spinal cord: dependence of the relative biological effectiveness on dose and linear energy transfer. Radiother Oncol 2015;117:358–363.

89 Warrington JP, Ashpole N, Csiszar A, Lee YW, Ungvari Z, Sonntag WE: Whole brain radiation-induced vascular cognitive impairment: mechanisms and implications. J Vasc Res 2013;50:445–457.

90 Cutter DJ, Schaapveld M, Darby SC, Hauptmann M, van Nimwegen FA, Krol ADG, et al: Risk for valvular heart disease after treatment for Hodgkin lymphoma. J Natl Cancer Inst 2015;107:1–9.

91 Darby SC, Ewertz M, McGale P, Bennet AM, Blom-Goldman U, Brønnum D, et al: Risk of ischemic heart disease in women after radiotherapy for breast cancer. N Engl J Med 2013;368:987–998.

92 Tapio S: Pathology and biology of radiation-induced cardiac disease. J Radiat Res 2016;57:439–448.

93 Wittig A, Engenhart-Cabillic R: Cardiac side effects of conventional and particle radiotherapy in cancer patients. Herz 2011;36:311–324.

94 Wang X, Zhang X, Li X, Amos RA, Shaitelman SF, Hoffman K, et al: Accelerated partial-breast irradiation using intensity-modulated proton radiotherapy: do uncertainties outweigh potential benefits? Br J Radiol 2013;86:20130176.

95 Bush DA, Slater JD, Garberoglio C, Do S, Lum S, Slater JM: Partial breast irradiation delivered with proton beam: results of a phase II trial. Clin Breast Cancer 2011;11:241–245.

96 Chang JH, Lee NK, Kim JY, Kim Y-J, Moon SH, Kim TH, et al: Phase II trial of proton beam accelerated partial breast irradiation in breast cancer. Radiother Oncol 2013;108:209–214.

97 Bert C, Engenhart-Cabillic R, Durante M: Particle therapy for noncancer diseases. Med Phys 2012;39:1716–1727.

98 Lehmann HI, Richter D, Prokesch H, Graeff C, Prall M, Simoniello P, et al: AV Node ablation in Langendorff-perfused porcine hearts using carbon ion particle therapy: methods and an in vivo feasibility investigation for catheter-free ablation of cardiac arrhythmias. Circ Arrhythmia Electrophysiol 2015;8:429–438.

99 Lehmann HI, Graeff C, Simoniello P, Constantinescu A, Takami M, Lugenbiel P, et al: Feasibility study on cardiac arrhythmia ablation using high-energy heavy ion beams. Sci Rep 2016;6:1–13.

100 Libby P, Ridker PM, Hansson GK: Progress and challenges in translating the biology of atherosclerosis. Nature 2011;473:317–325.

101 Tabas I, García-Cardeña G, Owens GK: Recent insights into the cellular biology of atherosclerosis. J Cell Biol 2015;209:13–22.

102 Hendry JH, Akahoshi M, Wang LS, Lipshultz SE, Stewart FA, Trott KR: Radiation-induced cardiovascular injury. Radiat Environ Biophys 2008;47:189–193.

103 Little MP, Gola A, Tzoulaki I: A model of cardiovascular disease giving a plausible mechanism for the effect of fractionated low-dose ionizing radiation exposure. PLoS Comput Biol 2009;5:e1000539.

104 Baselet B, Rombouts C, Benotmane A, Baatout S, Aerts A: Cardiovascular diseases related to ionizing radiation: the risk of low-dose exposure (review). Int J Mol Med 2016;38:1623–1641.

105 Mancuso M, Pasquali E, Braga-Tanaka I, Tanaka S, Pannicelli A, Giardullo P, et al: Acceleration of atherogenesis in ApoE⁻ᐟ⁻ mice exposed to acute or low-dose-rate ionizing radiation. Oncotarget 2015;6:31263–31271.

106 Yu T, Parks BW, Yu S, Srivastava R, Gupta K, Wu X, et al: Iron-ion radiation accelerates atherosclerosis in apolipoprotein E-deficient mice. Radiat Res 2011;175:766–773.

107 Aleman BMP, Moser EC, Nuver J, Suter TM, Maraldo M V, Specht L, et al: Cardiovascular disease after cancer therapy. EJC Suppl 2014;12:18–28.

108 Bakshi M V, Barjaktarovic Z, Azimzadeh O, Kempf SJ, Merl J, Hauck SM, et al: Long-term effects of acute low-dose ionizing radiation on the neonatal mouse heart: a proteomic study. Radiat Environ Biophys 2013;52:451–461.

109 Amino M, Yoshioka K, Tanabe T, Tanaka E, Mori H, Furusawa Y, et al: Heavy ion radiation up-regulates Cx43 and ameliorates arrhythmogenic substrates in hearts after myocardial infarction. Cardiovasc Res 2006;72:412–421.

110 Amino M, Yoshioka K, Fujibayashi D, Hashida T, Furusawa Y, Zareba W, et al: Year-long upregulation of connexin43 in rabbit hearts by heavy ion irradiation. Am J Physiol Heart Circ Physiol 2010;298:H1014–H1021.

111 Ghobadi G, van der Veen S, Bartelds B, de Boer RA, Dickinson MG, de Jong JR, et al: Physiological interaction of heart and lung in thoracic irradiation. Int J Radiat Oncol Biol Phys 2012;84:e639–e646.

112 Yarnold J, Vozenin Brotons M-C: Pathogenetic mechanisms in radiation fibrosis. Radiother Oncol 2010;97:149–161.

113 Fournier C, Scholz M, Weyrather WK, Rodemann HP, Kraft G: Changes of fibrosis-related parameters after high- and low-LET irradiation of fibroblasts. Int J Radiat Biol 2001;77:713–722.

114 Sorensen BS, Horsman MR, Alsner J, Overgaard J, Durante M, Scholz M, et al: Relative biological effectiveness of carbon ions for tumor control, acute skin damage and late radiation-induced fibrosis in a mouse model. Acta Oncol 2015;54:1623–1630.

115 Tinganelli W, Durante M, Helm A: Clinical evidence and radiobiological background of particle radiation therapy; in Pirtoli L, Gravina GL, Giordano A (eds): Radiobiology of Glioblastoma, ed 1. Cham, Springer International, 2016, pp 63–85.

116 Durante M, Tommasino F, Yamada S: Modeling combined chemotherapy and particle therapy for locally advanced pancreatic cancer. Front Oncol 2015;5:145.

117 Lock M, Muinuddin A, Kocha WI, Dinniwell R, Rodrigues G, D'souza D: Abscopal effects: case report and emerging opportunities. Cureus 2015;7:e344.

118 Durante M, Reppingen N, Held KD: Immunologically augmented cancer treatment using modern radiotherapy. Trends Mol Med 2013;19:565–582.

119 Formenti SC, Demaria S: Combining radiotherapy and cancer immunotherapy: a paradigm shift. J Natl Cancer Inst 2013;105:256–265.

120 Teng MWL, Galon J, Fridman WH, Smyth MJ: From mice to humans: developments in cancer immunoediting. J Clin Invest 2015;125:3338–3346.

121 Golden EB, Frances D, Pellicciotta I, Demaria S, Helen Barcellos-Hoff M, Formenti SC: Radiation fosters dose-dependent and chemotherapy-induced immunogenic cell death. Oncoimmunology 2014;3:e28518.

122 Finkelstein SE, Timmerman R, McBride WH, Schaue D, Hoffe SE, Mantz CA, et al: The confluence of stereotactic ablative radiotherapy and tumor immunology. Clin Dev Immunol 2011; 2011:439752.

123 Kim MS, Kim W, Park IH, Kim HJ, Lee E, Jung JH, et al: Radiobiological mechanisms of stereotactic body radiation therapy and stereotactic radiation surgery. Radiat Oncol J 2015;33:265–275.

124 Durante M, Brenner DJ, Formenti SC: Does heavy ion therapy work through the immune system? Int J Radiat Oncol Biol Phys 2016;96:934–936.

125 Gameiro SR, Malamas AS, Bernstein MB, Tsang KY, Vassantachart A, Sahoo N, et al: Tumor cells surviving exposure to proton or photon radiation share a common immunogenic modulation signature, rendering them more sensitive to T cell-mediated killing. Int J Radiat Oncol Biol Phys 2016;95:120–130.

126 Shimokawa T, Ma L, Ando K, Sato K, Imai T: The future of combining carbon-ion radiotherapy with immunotherapy: evidence and progress in mouse models. Int J Part Ther 2016;3:61–70.

127 Loeffler JS, Durante M: Charged particle therapy – optimization, challenges and future directions. Nat Rev Clin Oncol 2013;10:411–424.

128 Crittenden M, Kohrt H, Levy R, Jones J, Camphausen K, Dicker A, et al: Current clinical trials testing combinations of immunotherapy and radiation. Semin Radiat Oncol 2015;25:54–64.

129 Postow MA, Callahan MK, Barker CA, Yamada Y, Yuan J, Kitano S, et al: Immunologic correlates of the abscopal effect in a patient with melanoma. N Engl J Med 2012;366:925–931.

130 Garcia-Barros M, Paris F, Cordon-Cardo C, Lyden D, Rafii S, Haimovitz-Friedman A, et al: Tumor response to radiotherapy regulated by endothelial cell apoptosis. Science 2003;300:1155–1159.

131 Kolesnick R, Fuks Z: Radiation and ceramide-induced apoptosis. Oncogene 2003;22:5897–5906.

132 Corre I, Guillonneau M, Paris F: Membrane signaling induced by high doses of ionizing radiation in the endothelial compartment: relevance in radiation toxicity. Int J Mol Sci 2013;14:22678–22696.

133 Helm A, Lee R, Durante M, Ritter S: The influence of C-ions and X-rays on human umbilical vein endothelial cells. Front Oncol 2016;6:5.

134 Grabham P, Hu B, Sharma P, Geard C: Effects of ionizing radiation on three-dimensional human vessel models: differential effects according to radiation quality and cellular development. Radiat Res 2011;175:21–28.

135 Seideman JH, Stancevic B, Rotolo JA, McDevitt MR, Howell RW, Kolesnick RN, et al: Alpha particles induce apoptosis through the sphingomyelin pathway. Radiat Res 2011;176:434–446.

136 Alphonse G, Maalouf M, Battiston-Montagne P, Ardail D, Beuve M, Rousson R, et al: P53-independent early and late apoptosis is mediated by ceramide after exposure of tumor cells to photon or carbon ion irradiation. BMC Cancer 2013;13:151.

137 Laine AM, Pompos A, Timmerman R, Jiang S, Story MD, Pistenmaa D, et al: The role of hypofractionated radiation therapy with photons, protons, and heavy ions for treating extracranial lesions. Front Oncol 2016;5:302.

Marco Durante
Trento Institute for Fundamental Physics and Applications-National Institute for Nuclear Physics (TIFPA-INFN)
University of Trento
Via Sommarive 14, IT–38121 Trento (Italy)
E-Mail marco.durante@tifpa.infn.it

Guckenberger M, Combs SE, Zips D (eds): Advances in Radiotherapy.
Prog Tumor Res. Basel, Karger, 2018, vol 44, pp 122–129 (DOI: 10.1159/000486999)

Preclinical Mouse Models for the Evaluation of Novel Techniques in Particle Therapy

Thomas Ernst Schmid · Gabriele Multhoff

Department of Radiation Oncology and Center for Translational Cancer Research (TranslaTUM), Klinikum rechts der Isar, Technische Universität München, Munich, and Institute of Innovative Radiotherapy, Helmholtz Zentrum München, Neuherberg, Germany

Abstract

Preclinical mouse models that allow the evaluation of novel techniques in radiotherapy using charged particles like protons or heavier ions are discussed here. Focused beams of protons or carbon ions offer distinct physical characteristics that might contribute to an overall improved risk-benefit profile in radiotherapy. In the last decade, novel concepts in radiotherapy aimed to optimize the delivery of high radiation doses to the tumor while sparing the surrounding healthy tissue. 2D in vitro tumor cell cultures provide experimental models to determine the radiosensitivity of isolated cells to different radiation qualities. However, these cell culture models are not capable of mimicking the complexity and heterogeneity of 3-dimensionally growing clinical tumors with their individual tumor microenvironment. Therefore, small animal tumor models are urgently needed to study radiation responses after particle radiotherapy in vivo. Here we describe the recent developments and the accurate testing of novel techniques in particle radiotherapy using up-to-date preclinical animal models.

The focus of this article is preclinical models for the evaluation of novel techniques in radiotherapy using charged particles like protons or heavy ions. The use of particle radiotherapy, in particular proton and carbon ion radiation, has grown in the last decade because of its improved ability to minimize radiation-induced damage in the surrounding normal tissues. Minimizing normal tissue damage is particularly important when tumors are localized in close proximity to radiation-sensitive critical structures, such as the brain, spinal cord, heart, stomach, and small bowel [1]. Today, beams of protons or heavy ions, predominantly carbon ions, can be accelerated to precisely calculated energies, which can be accurately targeted to tumors. Particle irradiation offers distinct physical characteristics that contribute to an overall improved risk-benefit profile in radiotherapy. The superior in-depth dose distribution of particles allows a more precise dose administration, resulting in an increased therapeutic ratio [2]. This increased therapeutic ratio may also permit dose escalation to the tumor and therefore might result in a better tumor control. Particle irradiation with high linear energy transfer (LET) offers additional increased radiobiological efficacy, especially with respect to the Bragg peak [3]. This radiobiological difference could decrease the influence of the cell cycle phase as well as the oxygenation in tumor radiotherapy. In the last decade, novel techniques in radiotherapy have focused mainly on optimizing the delivery of a high radiation dose to the tumor while sparing the surrounding healthy tissue. The development and implementation of novel techniques in radiotherapy necessitates accurate testing in preclinical animal models. However, in the last decade most studies were performed in 2D cell culture systems, and the number of in vivo studies in radiotherapy has remained limited in recent decades.

Preclinical Models for Particle Radiotherapy

2D tumor cell cultures provide experimental models to determine tumor cell viability after exposure to different radiation qualities. The clonogenic cell survival assay, which measures the clonogenic capacity of individual tumor cells to grow under cell culture conditions, has so far been the gold standard for determining radiosensitivity [4]. The assay essentially tests the ability of a singular tumor cell to undergo "unlimited" division under homogenous 2D culture conditions [5]. Also, the effects of protons or heavy ions can be determined by the clonogenic cell survival assay. The effect of particle irradiation has been evaluated in a range of in vitro studies, demonstrating an increased relative biological effectiveness (RBE) with an increasing LET, as reviewed by Friedrich et al. [6] and Elsasser et al. [7].

However, these conventional 2D cell cultures are not capable of mimicking the complexity of tumors as in vivo tumors grow 3-dimensionally and, depending on the tumor microenvironment, the tumors show a high grade of heterogeneity. The main limitation of 2D tumor cell cultures is the wrong assumption that all tumor cells are identical in a 3D tumor in vivo. Therefore, tumor cell lines are not representative for primary tumors in vivo. In line with this hypothesis, the study by Shai et al. [8] demonstrated that tumor cells grown for only 3 passages in cell culture no longer represented the cellular composition of the original tumor from which they were derived. Moreover, in vitro cell cultures lack the cellular complexity of in vivo tumors because they do not account for inflammatory or vascular components [4].

The most simple model for investigating the radiation response after photon or particle radiotherapy in vivo is an ectopic xenograft model which involves the subcutaneous injection of viable human tumor cells into the hind leg or back of immunocompromised mice or rats [9]. In cases where the immune system of the immunocompromised small animals does not allow the growth of xenograft human tumors, it is recommendable to perform a whole body irradiation at 2–4 Gy approximately 24 h before tumor cell inoculation. A major advantage of a subcutaneous tumor mouse model is the possibility to measure tumor growth regularly and with minimal invasive methods, such as a caliper or by ultrasound technique.

If factors of the tumor microenvironment are essential for the growth of a certain tumor type, orthotopic xenograft models should be used. A major advantage of orthotopic tumor models is the possibility to induce metastatic dissemination of the tumor like in the original human primary tumor. As an example, human breast carcinoma cells that are implanted into the fat mammary tissue of immune-deficient mice can induce metastases in the lung, liver, and brain, similar to human breast carcinoma patients. Disadvantages of orthotopic xenograft mouse models involve complex surgeries under aesthesis, difficulties in tumor imaging, and negative side effects on the organ function of the implanted mice and rats. Today, in vivo imaging methods are frequently applied to monitor tumor growth in orthotopic animal models. Especially in vivo targeting of tumors using tumor-specific fluorescently labeled or radiolabeled probes have greatly gained in importance over the last few years [10].

It is important to note that xenograft tumor models using human tumor cell lines have only a limited clinical relevance in judging the response of a patient's tumor to a certain particular radiation treatment. To overcome this limitation, small (1 mm^3) cubes of freshly isolated patient-derived tumor material can also be used for the transplantation into immune-compromised mice [11]. However, due to limitations in cell viability in solid tumor tissues, the take rate of patient-derived tumor xenografts is frequently less than 25%. The whole body irradiation of immune-compromised mice can further enhance the tumor take of patient-derived tumor biopsy material. Despite these problems patient-derived tumor xenografts are certainly an extremely promising model for personalized cancer therapy [11].

However, all human tumor xenograft models are limited by the lack of an individual immune system in the mice. This means that the lymphocyte-mediated immune responses to the tumor are lacking because athymic nude mice have no mature T cells and SCID/bg mice are lacking functional T, B, and NK cells.

To overcome these limitations regarding the impact of the host's immune system, syngeneic mouse tumor models can be used. Syngeneic tumor models involve tumor cells derived from the same genetic background of a given inbred mouse strain. The main advantage of syngeneic models is that the host immune system is active, and thus better represents the tumor microenvironment of a patient's tumor. A disadvantage of these syngeneic tumor mouse models relates to the fact that immune cells in humans and mice are different.

Therefore, rodent tumor cells as compared to human cells are less effective in the activation of checkpoint inhibitor blockades, or have a higher sensitivity towards oxidative stress [4, 12, 13]. Furthermore, drugs as well as cytokines can be species specific, and thus do not properly reflect the human situation. Due to these differences between rodent and human cells, most preclinical radiation studies frequently focus on human tumor xenografts [4].

Most similarities to the human tumor situation are reflected by spontaneous or genetically engineered tumor mouse models, such as the colitis-associated spontaneous tumor model, as described by Greten et al. [14], or the endogenous pancreatic ductal and lung adenocarcinoma mouse models [15]. The latter pancreatic ductal adenocarcinoma model involves genetic modifications in Kras, p53, and CKP, which are resembled by human tumors. Although these models have a high clinical relevance, they are hampered by the fact that tumors in mice occur only rarely, it takes several months to obtain measurable tumors, and the frequent use of imaging techniques is necessary to find the tumor location [16–19].

Preclinical Evaluation for the Optimization of Carbon Ion Radiotherapy

Tumor growth delay as an endpoint using carbon ion radiation has been the focus of a range of studies comparing carbon ions (high-LET) with photons (low-LET). Tumor growth delay is a popular endpoint in radiotherapy of mouse tumor models and is defined as the difference between the mean time nonirradiated tumors needed to reach 5 times their volume and the mean time irradiated tumors needed to reach 5 times the volume at the time of irradiation.

The study by Ando et al. [20] compared the RBE between the tumor growth delay and an early skin reaction of syngeneic mice. The investigators treated fibrosarcoma xenografts and host mouse skin with γ-rays or carbon ion beams with 3 different LET values (20, 42, and 77 keV/μm) and with 1–7 fractions. They could demonstrate that the RBE was higher for a tumor than for skin after carbon ion irradiation. The therapeutic gain, which was calculated as the ratio of the RBE value for tumor growth delay to that for early skin reaction, was highest when the radiation was performed in 4 fractions. The study by Takahashi et al. [21] measured the RBE of carbon-ion beams on tumor growth delay of esophageal tumors in mice. The study indicated that carbon ions are more effective than photon irradiation. The RBE of carbon ions against X-rays was 2.02. Another tumor growth delay study performed by Yoshida et al. [22] used C-ion radiotherapy beams in 1–12 fractions separated by 4 h in transplanted fibrosarcoma tumors. The authors demonstrated that higher doses per fraction are suitable for C-ion radiotherapy irrespective of LET.

However, to date, only a very limited number of in vivo studies have focused on tumor control. The study by Sorenson et al. [46] compared the biological effectiveness of carbon ions relative to X-rays for tumor control in CDF1 mice with a C3H mouse mammary carcinoma implanted subcutaneously on the foot of the right hind limb. The RBE for tumor control was only 1.48 [17]. In contrast, in the study by Peschke et al. [47], an RBE of 2.3 was found in a radioresistant rat prostate tumor (Dunning subline R3327-AT1); the mean dose-averaged LET was approximately 75 keV/μm, with 1 fraction [15, 16]. However, due to the low number of in vivo studies conducted so far, the effect of carbon ion dose fractionation in different tumors and normal tissues in the same mouse model should be further investigated and the factors that can affect the results of fractionated irradiation (e.g., hypoxia, cell cycle, and DNA repair capacity) should be considered [23].

The nervous system is critical for toxicity because of the low capacity for regeneration [23].

The sensitivity of the central nervous system to carbon ions has been examined in multiple experimental models. Yoshida et al. [24] used 10-day-old rats to assess any morphological changes and cellular apoptosis. The authors found that the RBE value for rat cerebellum was between 1.4 and 1.5. A study by Al-Jahdari et al. [25] investigated the sensitivity of the peripheral nervous system to carbon ions, which resulted in an RBE value of 3.1–3.2 in day 8 neurons and 1.5–2.1 in day 16 neurons. It is known that the RBE value for carbon ions in tumor radiotherapy is normally between 2 and 3, and these findings suggest a wider therapeutic window for carbon ions than for X-rays for the treatment of tumors next to the central or peripheral nervous system [23].

Radiosensitizers can improve radiotherapy by sensitizing tumor cells to radiation, thereby achieving the similar effects with a lower radiation dose. To date, there have been many reports of radiosensitizers for photon irradiation, but only a few studies on radiosensitizers for carbon-ion radiotherapy. The study by Hirakawa et al. [26] analyzed tumor growth delay of SQ5 human lung tumor cells using a mouse xenograft model after 17-allylamino-17-demethoxygeldanamycin (17-AAG) pretreatment and carbon ion irradiation. The findings demonstrated that the combination of high-LET carbon ion irradiation and an Hsp90 inhibitor leads to an improved tumor growth delay.

Preclinical Evaluation of Spatial Fractionation for Particle Therapy

It is well known that particle radiation therapy has important advantages compared with photons with respect to the dose distribution in the depth of the tissue, which can limit the dose to the normal tissue [27]. On the other hand, particle irradiation with protons and heavy ions still causes normal tissue damage, which can lead to

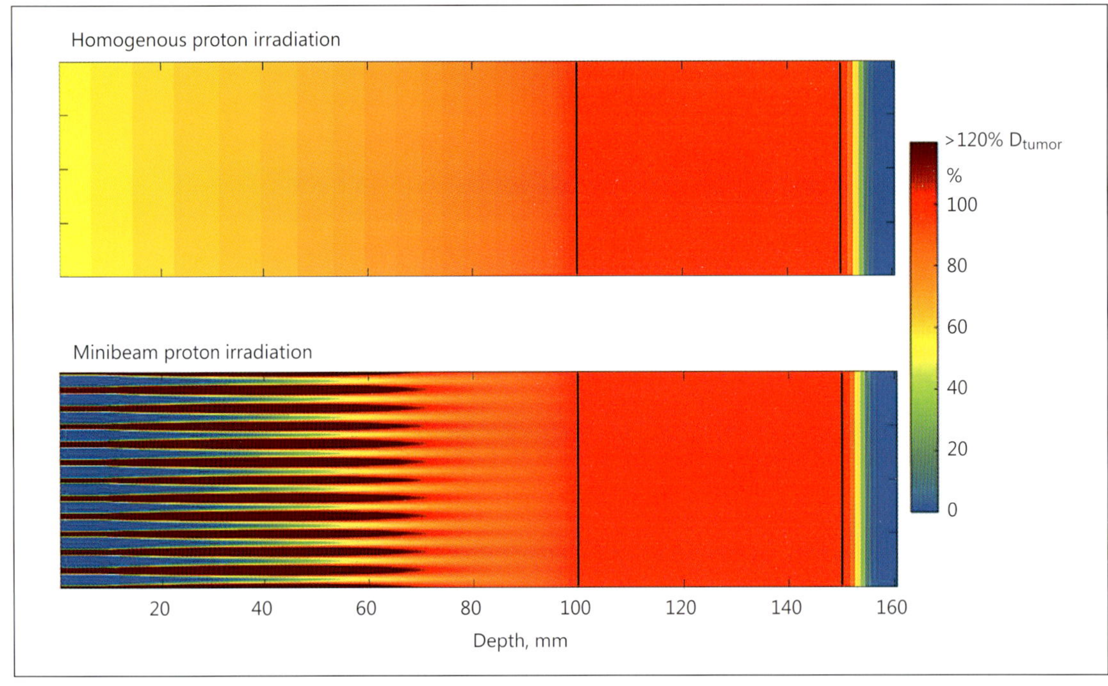

Fig. 1. Simulated dose distributions for homogeneous broad beam and minibeam.

acute or late radiation effects and which can also induce the development of secondary cancer, with detrimental effects on the patient's well-being after radiation therapy. New technologies, such as microbeam radiation therapy (MRT), which was developed at Brookhaven National Laboratory [28] and the European Synchrotron Radiation Facility [29–31], have shown increased normal tissue preservation due to spatial fractionation. An innovative radiotherapy approach combines the advantages of both – protons and MRT – as an innovative strategy to limit the acute and late side effects of the radiotherapy. The technique is called proton minibeam radiation therapy and was developed at the ion microprobe SNAKE (superconducting nanoprobe for applied nuclear [Kern] physics experiments) in Munich [32–34].

Proton minibeam radiotherapy uses spatial fractionation, similar to MRT, with the aim of reducing normal tissue damage in the entrance channel. For this novel technique, submillimeter-sized proton beams spread with increasing track length due to interactions with the traversed tissue, which will finally lead to a homogeneous dose distribution inside the tumor (Fig. 1). The first experimental evidence of reduced normal tissue damage was shown in an in vitro 3D human skin model [34]. The study showed higher cell viability by the MTT test as well as lower cytogenetic damage by the micronuclei assay, together with a reduced inflammatory response, measured as the release of inflammatory cytokines in the culture medium [34]. The first in vivo study was performed by Girst et al. [35] in 2016, where minibeam and homogeneous irradiation was compared in a tumor-free mouse ear model to analyze acute normal tissue side effects, which takes into account the complex effects on the immune system and vasculature. The study demonstrated that proton minibeam radiation therapy results in reduced side effects compared with conventional

Schmid · Multhoff

broad-beam irradiation. Another study demonstrated the feasibility of the technical implementation of minibeam radiation therapy by experimental dosimetry [36]. The authors concluded that an array of 100-MeV proton minibeams could be used to treat a tumor in the center of the brain with a homogeneous dose distribution, while the normal tissues benefit from the spatial dose fractionation.

Similar approaches using minibeams for heavy ion therapy, for example carbon ions, might also be beneficial; however, the size of the minibeams would be smaller compared with those of protons due to the limited lateral spreading of heavier ions [35]. Minibeam irradiation with protons or heavy ions might be an innovative technique of particle radiotherapy that can further reduce the acute and late side effects of particle irradiations. However, more preclinical experiments are needed in order to evaluate the potential of this new technique.

Preclinical Evaluation of Laser-Driven Particle Acceleration

Due to the high cost of conventional accelerators, so far only a small number of ion beam facilities are in use worldwide. The potential advantages of laser-driven particle therapy arise from combining a compact, cost-efficient treatment unit with the physical advantages in the dose delivery of charged particle beams [37]. In the last decade, laser-driven charged particle acceleration has evolved quickly, and this promising new technology for particle radiation therapy could lead to lower treatment costs compared to conventional acceleration systems. However, one of the key differences with regard to radiobiological properties of laser-accelerated particles is that laser-driven particle beams are delivered in ultrashort pulses. While the duration of laser pulses is in the range of femtoseconds, the resulting particle pulse is in the nanosecond range because of spreading in time during beam transport [38]. In contrast,

conventional proton irradiation using cyclotrons or synchrotrons deliver the same dose over a time period of milliseconds to seconds, which is a difference of 6–9 orders of magnitude. Therefore, preclinical experiments are necessary to understand whether an ultra-high dose rate alters any relevant biological endpoints. In the last decade, several experiments explored different endpoints in vitro, like DNA repair, cytogenetic damage, and cell death in monolayer cell cultures using the ultra-high dose rates [39–42]. However, these studies showed no indication for a significantly altered radiobiology of pulsed protons at ultra-high dose rates in vitro. Also, data from first radiobiological in vitro experiments with laser-driven protons and electrons revealed no differences with respect to the RBE values compared to conventional irradiation sources [43]. In experiments using laser-accelerated 5-MeV protons [44], the biological response in terms of initial damage to the deoxyribonucleic acid (DNA) was quantified using the g-H2AX assay. The RBE obtained in this study is in agreement with proton RBE values in conventional beams at comparable proton energy [44].

In 2012, a technical set-up (Fig. 2) for in vivo irradiation of subcutaneous tumors in mice was constructed and successfully tested using a mouse xenograft tumor model [45]. For these experiments, human-derived head and neck squamous cell carcinoma FaDu was cut into small pieces and transplanted subcutaneously into the left hind leg of anaesthetized mice. The animals were subjected to proton irradiation as soon as the tumors had reached a maximum size of 4 mm in depth, as determined by daily ultrasound measurements. This was the first step towards a preclinical platform for high-precision image-guided particle therapy for radiobiological research in small animals. Only 2 years later, in the first in vivo study, FaDu tumors in the hind leg of a mouse were irradiated using 20 Gy of 23-MeV protons with single pulses of 1 ns duration or in a continuous mode (100 ms), and the tumor growth delay was